# The SKINNY on FATS

David Brownstein, M.D. & Sheryl Shenefelt, C.N.

For further copies of *The Skinny on Fats:*

Order online: www.drbrownstein.com or www.sherylshenefelt.com

Call: 1-888-647-5616 or send a check or money order in the amount of: $23.00 ($18.00 plus $5.00 shipping and handling) or for Michigan residents $24.08 ($18.00 plus $5.00 shipping and handling, plus $1.08 sales tax) to:

Healthy Living
964 Floyd Street
Birmingham, Michigan 48009

The Skinny on Fats, 1st Edition


ISBN: 978-0-9840869-2-4
Healthy Living
964 Floyd Street
Birmingham, Michigan 48009
(248) 851-3372
(888) 647-5616

Center for Holistic Medicine
(248) 851-1600

# Acknowledgements


## David Brownstein, M.D.

I gratefully acknowledge the help I have received from my friends and colleagues in putting this book together. This book could not have been published without help from the editors—my wife Allison and Janet Darnell.

I would also like to thank my patients. It is your search for safe and effective natural treatments that is the driving force behind holistic medicine. You have accompanied me down this path and I appreciate each and every one of you.

And, to my staff. Thank you so very much for taking this trip with me. Without your help and support, none of this would be possible. I do appreciate all of your hard work and your dedication.

## Sheryl Shenefelt, C.N.

I am extremely grateful for all of the help and support I received from my family and friends as well as my newsletter, blog, and Facebook community in putting this book together. I am so glad I connected with the Weston A. Price Foundation in the beginning of my journey learning about real food and real fats and their importance in a healthy diet. I am thankful to Dr. David Brownstein for the opportunity to write our fifth book together and I look forward to our continued relationship.

I also appreciate the editing guidance from Lisa Howard and Jan Darnell as well as reviewing and support from Angelle Batten, Angela Biggs, Ann Salomon and Allison Selko. Finally, to my three favorite people in the whole world: my husband Bob, daughter Grace, and son Nicholas. I am forever grateful to you for your love, patience, and ongoing encouragement as I continue to write about and share with the world about real food, nutrition, and how to be healthy!

## A Word of Caution to the Reader

The information presented in this book is based on the training and professional experience of the authors. The advice in this book should not be undertaken without first consulting a physician. Proper laboratory and clinical monitoring is essential to achieving the goals of finding safe and effective natural treatments. This book was written for informational and educational purposes only. It is not intended to be used as medical advice.

# Dedications

***David Brownstein, M.D.***

*To the women of my life: Allison, Hailey, and Jessica, with all my love.*

*And, to my patients. Thank you for being interested in what I am interested in.*

***Sheryl Shenefelt, C.N.***

*With love to my wonderful husband Bob and beautiful children Grace and Nicholas.*

# Contents

# Preface

## David Brownstein, M.D.

In medical school, I was instructed that everybody needs to reduce dietary fat. Furthermore, I was told that all saturated fat products caused heart disease and that a low-fat diet was the best diet for everyone. Looking back on what I was taught in medical school amazes me. Why? Because so much of what I was taught was wrong.

I graduated from medical school right in the middle of the low-fat dietary craze. There were low-fat choices for so many food products. People would proudly state that they ate a low-fat diet. I bought into the low-fat dietary advice since that was what I was taught.

However, when I decided to look outside of what I learned in medical school, things began to change. I began to practice holistic medicine after discovering why my father was suffering from heart disease. My father, Ellis, had his first heart attack at age 40 and a second myocardial infarction at age 42. Over the next 20 years, he had coronary bypass surgeries, coronary angioplasties, and was treated with over 12 different medications to treat high cholesterol, diabetes, and hypertension. When I finished my medical training, I read a book titled, *Healing With Nutrition.* In this book, the author, my friend and mentor, Dr. Jonathan Wright wrote that heart disease is not caused by a lack of cardiac medications. Rather it is caused by an imbalance of the hormonal and nutritional systems. When I looked at my father in this manner, I quickly discovered he was lacking basic nutrients and was hormonally imbalanced. I placed him initially on two natural items: natural testosterone and natural thyroid hormone. Within four weeks, his 20 year history of angina went away, never to return. Also, during this same time, his cholesterol levels fell below 200mg/dl—they had always been over 300mg/dl. Most importantly, my father looked and acted better. Once I saw the changes in my father, I knew that I needed to change my practice to a more holistic practice.

My father was not the best patient. He ate too much food and liked rich, sugary products. But, on the advice of his physicians, he would always choose low-fat food items. I began to check my father's various nutrient levels and discovered that he was deficient in all the fat-soluble vitamins and that his fatty acid profile was also imbalanced.

Once I began changing my practice philosophy, I realized that I had to address my patients' dietary habits. In reading about various diets, I began to realize that, for the answer to the question "What is a healthy diet?", my medical training was inadequate. When I looked at the research, I found that there were no credible studies showing that a low-fat diet was beneficial for anyone. In fact, once I began to dissect the dietary studies, I found harm with low-fat diets. In fact, low-fat diets make neither biochemical nor common sense. I realized that low-fat diets lead to many health problems including fatigue, cancer, brain disorders, fibromyalgia, and even cardiovascular disease. My research led me to conclude that low-fat diets were harmful.

I studied the research from many prominent doctors. Dr. Weston A. Price had the largest influence on me. I read his book, *Nutrition and Physical Degeneration,* twice. Dr. Price travelled the world and found the healthiest cultures ate adequate amounts of fat (including saturated fat) in their diets. Once I started testing my patients for their nutritional status, I quickly realized Dr. Price was right; human beings require healthy fats in their diets. Since then, I have attended many seminars from the Weston A. Price Foundation. I would highly recommend these courses as a good way to gain dietary and nutritional knowledge.

I had my father alter his diet. He started adding eggs and healthy sources of fat in his diet. He began to eat fat from organic animal sources. I told him to avoid all low-fat food products—just as I advise my patients to do now.

My father, like everyone else who follows this advice, enjoyed his food much more. More importantly, he became healthier.

*The Skinny on Fats* was written to educate you about fat and dispel the myths about fat. You don't need to fear dietary fat, you just need to be educated about which forms of dietary fat are the healthiest. *The Skinny on Fats* will provide you with that information.

Low-fat diets are not only unhealthy, they are dangerous. I am sure when you read what Sheryl and I have to say about dietary fat, you will come to the same conclusion that we have.

David Brownstein, M.D. 5.1.14
www.drbrownstein.com

## Sheryl Shenefelt, C.N.

"Avoid fat." "Eat low-fat." "Fat will make you fat." "High cholesterol causes heart disease." This is what we have been told for decades through almost all mainstream media sources, dieticians and physicians. When people come to see me for nutrition advice they have what I call "fat phobia." They believe that in order to be healthy and to lose weight they need to avoid fat at all costs. Of course, they have also wrongly been led to believe they must stay away from saturated fats and instead choose fats that are labeled as "heart-healthy" and "low in cholesterol." It's time for people to learn the truth about fats. Also, it is time to learn that saturated fat has been wrongly lumped together with the truly bad fats: trans fats. The real message is that optimal health is not possible without eating adequate amounts of good fats, including saturated fat!

The goal I had for writing this book with Dr. Brownstein was to explain why we need fat not only to live, but to thrive. We see countless people who are eating low-fat diets and wondering why they do not feel healthier. Many of them are severely nutrient-deficient, unhappy, and overweight. Many people are confused about fats. Looking to the media, dieticians, or even our own doctors is not the answer. They will feed you the same story that fat is bad for you and you should avoid it.

This book was written to help you shift your paradigms about fat. This book will help you realize that low-fat, high-carb diets are **not** the answer. Furthermore, avoiding fat is not the way to lose weight. In fact, some of the very fats we have been told to avoid—coconut oil being a prime example—can actually boost metabolism and lead to weight loss. Adding fat to your diet will help you feel happier and healthier. Use the recipes and the *Know Your Fats Quick Reference Guide* in the back of the book to help you get started.

The standard American diet (SAD) consists of too many high-carb and processed foods–that's the kind found in boxes, bags, cans, and packages. These foods contain too little good-quality fat (although they do contain plenty of the bad and ugly fats we discuss in this book).

And not only are processed foods high in sugar and lacking in good fats, they are also lacking in other vital nutrients such as vitamins, minerals, and enzymes. Examples of these poor-quality foods include food that has been sweetened (both artificially and with refined sugar), food containing refined vegetable oils, hydrogenated oils or trans fats, food that has been stripped of nutrients, food that has been overheated or chemically treated, and foods containing preservatives, stabilizers, artificial colors and flavors. In other words, processed foods are devitalized "non-foods" which are devoid of nutrients—instead, they contain bad fats, sugars, and anti-nutrients that harm normal brain and body functions. These are the true enemies and contributors to chronic illnesses such as heart disease and cancer.

We wrote this book to give you the real skinny on fat and also teach you which types of fat are healthy for the body and which types of fat should be avoided. Some of them will doubtless be a surprise to you after all the misguided messages you've received about fat!

Be Well!

Sheryl Shenefelt, C.N.
www.sherylshenefelt.com

# Introduction

**What if you found out** that healthy fat is not what causes obesity?

What if you realized you could eat fat **and** still lose weight?

What if you discovered that low-fat diets may be the leading contributor to depression, behavioral/psychological problems, and fatigue?

What if you found out that research does **not** support the purported link between saturated fat intake and heart disease and cancer?

What if you realized that cholesterol is actually a **protective** substance in the body?

What if you found out heart patients can have either high or low cholesterol and that cholesterol levels are irrelevant?

What if you discovered statins do **not** decrease mortality?

*For over 60 years, the battle cry of mainstream doctors and dieticians has been "Don't eat fat!" Conventional medicine declared that dietary fat was the cause of heart disease, obesity, chronic illness, and cancer. They concluded that Americans needed to lower their intake of dietary fat and cholesterol in order to be healthy.*

The media eagerly repeated these falsehoods about fat and cholesterol and spread the low-fat mantra. The American Diabetic Association, the American Heart Association, and the American Academy of Nutrition and Dietetics (formally the American Dietetic Association) as well as other mainstream medical associations all told us the same message: "We must lower our dietary fat intake." So, what did we do? Over the last 60 years, we followed their advice and lowered our dietary fat intake. Are we healthier for it? Have obesity rates gone down? Do we enjoy lower rates of heart disease, chronic illness or cancer because we're eating less fat? The answer to all of these questions is a resounding "No."

We have been brainwashed into thinking that a low-fat diet is a healthy diet. If a low-fat diet is the answer, then why haven't rates of obesity and heart disease decreased in conjunction with our decreased rates of dietary fat intake? If a low-fat diet is the answer, why are over 97 million Americans (one-third of the population) struggling with obesity? Why is heart disease still one of the top killers in the U.S.?

The reason we are not seeing health benefits from a low-fat diet is that the message we've been getting for over 60 years is wrong. Far from being a dietary demon, fat is a vital and an essential part of our diet. In fact, we cannot live without adequate amounts of dietary fat, including saturated fat and cholesterol.

Low-fat and low-cholesterol diets are not healthy. They can lead to vitamin and mineral deficiencies, immune dysfunction, and hormonal issues, as well as other problems including degenerative diseases. What **is** healthy are adequate levels of healthy dietary fat, as well as sufficient amounts of whole-food sources that contain protein, fat, and carbohydrates along with essential vitamins and minerals. Fat and cholesterol are especially important for babies and children whose developing brains require healthy fats (and cholesterol) for normal brain development. It is important to note that fat is the most concentrated form of energy available to our bodies. It also provides the building blocks for cell membranes and a variety of hormones and hormone-like substances. Fat also helps the body absorb both vitamins and minerals from the diet. And those are just a few of the benefits of fat! You'll learn about many other amazing attributes of fat in this book.

That said, not all fat is good for us. Many fats—especially the refined, hydrogenated, and rancid fats found in many processed foods and in many restaurants—are harmful. So, which fats are good? Which are bad? In this book, we'll give you the skinny on fat and show you which types of fat are healthy and which types should be avoided.

When two-thirds of our adult population is overweight and the other third is obese, something isn't right. Low-fat diets are not the answer! In fact, they are one of the main causes of the obesity epidemic. We firmly believe that the rising rates of obesity and associated metabolic disorders (such as type II diabetes, cancer, and heart disease) are a direct result of following low-fat dietary recommendations. By the time you've finished reading this book, it should not shock you when we say that Americans need to avoid low-fat diets and reintroduce healthy fats back onto our plates.

Low-fat diets lead to deficiencies of essential fatty acids (e.g., omega-3 and omega-6 fats) as well as fat-soluble vitamins A, D, E, and K. Without adequate amounts of healthy dietary fat, we become undernourished and develop a host of age-related problems. Weight loss becomes difficult on a low-fat diet. As we will discuss further in Chapter 8, this is because when the body is starving for nutrients it will try to hold onto fat. Also, to achieve weight loss, we need to feel satiated, or we will continue to be plagued with hunger cravings that will cause us to overeat. At meal time, fat is what tells us that we're full because fat is what gives us the feeling of satiety. Did you know that optimal amounts of dietary fats are so necessary for our bodies to function that our bodies will lower our metabolism if we don't eat enough fat? Fat—not carbohydrates—is the preferred fuel for the human metabolism.

We wrote *The Skinny on Fats* to educate you about the importance of consuming good sources of dietary fats. This book will teach you why we need fat and why we can't live without it. It will also show you that high-carbohydrate, low-fat diets are the **root cause** of the obesity and chronic illness epidemics that we are facing. We contend that when you start adding more fats—the good fats—into your diet, you'll lose those extra pounds and feel healthier.

It's time for new dietary advice! This book will provide you with a new approach to food, fat, and health. Adopting the recommendations in this book will help you achieve and maintain your optimal health.

# 1

# The Fat Paradigm

# Fat makes us fat…or does it?

**Two-thirds of Americans are overweight** and over one-third are obese. Over 12.5 million children and teens are obese. Tragically, during the past 20 years, there has been a dramatic increase in obesity in the United States.[1] If we believe mainstream media, that's because we eat too much fat. But is that the truth?

For over 60 years, dieticians, mainstream medical doctors, the American Heart Association, the American Diabetes Association, American Academy of Nutrition and Dietetics (formerly the American Dietetic Association), as well as the rest of "The-Powers-That-Be" have all been preaching that we need to eat less fat. These groups all say the same thing: we are suffering a myriad of medical issues because we eat too much fat. These groups promised us that if we lowered our fat intake, we would have better health. We've done that. So what has happened over the last 60 years? By nearly every health indicator, we are moving in the wrong direction—we now have more obesity-related illnesses than we know what to do with.

Our paradigm about fat—specifically, the belief that we should all pursue low-fat diets—is based on outdated and unsubstantiated studies. One of the most influential authors of these studies was Ancel Keys, who told us that if we eat too much saturated fat we would clog our arteries, raise our cholesterol, and suffer from heart disease. We were told to eat foods labeled as "heart-healthy" and "low in cholesterol" because the fats these foods contained would not clog our arteries or make us get fat. This theory was a bad idea when it was born and a bad idea when it was implemented. It would be a **good** idea to put this theory to rest! We will discuss the diet/heart theory further in Chapter 2.

This anti-dietary fat paradigm is also reflected in the United States Department of Agriculture (USDA) official dietary guidelines. You can probably recall the food pyramid you learned in elementary school. We were taught that to be healthy, we should eat foods recommended by that pyramid. The original version recommended that we base our eating on carbohydrate sources and that we should limit fats and oils. This pyramid is depicted in Figure 1.

**Figure 1**

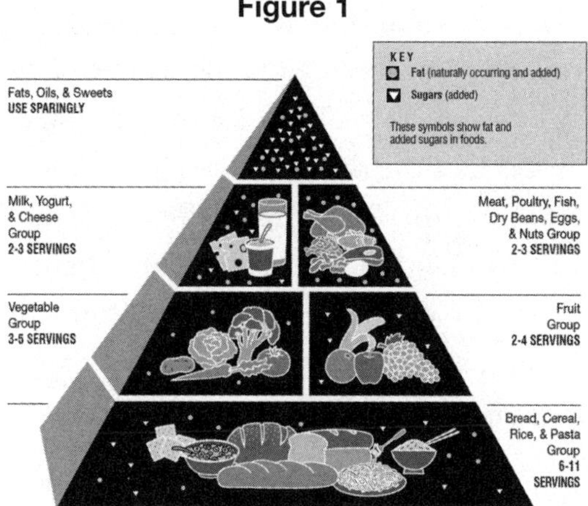


Today, the food pyramid has morphed into a food plate (MyPlate™), yet still has many of the same flaws that have existed since the first food pyramid was released. The USDA food plate still wrongly suggests that we increase our intake of carbohydrates and decrease our intake of fats and cholesterol-rich foods. See Figure 2 for the current MyPlate™.

What is wrong with the USDA food plate? After all, the new MyPlate™ was created to be an easily understood way to know what to eat. Unfortunately, because MyPlate™ will be so easily understood, more people will likely be following the **bad** advice it offers. Let's take a closer look at what's on our supposedly healthy plate now.

First of all, fats are not shown on the plate at all. What we do see is that at least half of our dietary intake should come from starches and sugars (grains and fruit), less than ¼ comes from protein and another ¼ comes from vegetables (which also could be starchy). Moreover, there is still no differentiation between "good proteins" and "bad proteins", "good carbs" and "bad carbs", or "good fats" and "bad fats".

But has the food pyramid/plate and the low-fat campaign influenced American's dietary choices? You better believe they have (and still do). We've spent the past 60 years listening to the USDA and The-Powers-That-Be and have obediently eaten less dietary fat, particularly fat from animal sources. Similarly, following the food pyramid/plate's guidelines, we've increased our intake of carbohydrates in the form of more grains. And we've changed our fat intake by avoiding saturated fat and increasing consumption of polyunsaturated fats such as vegetable oils and spreads.

**FIGURE 2**

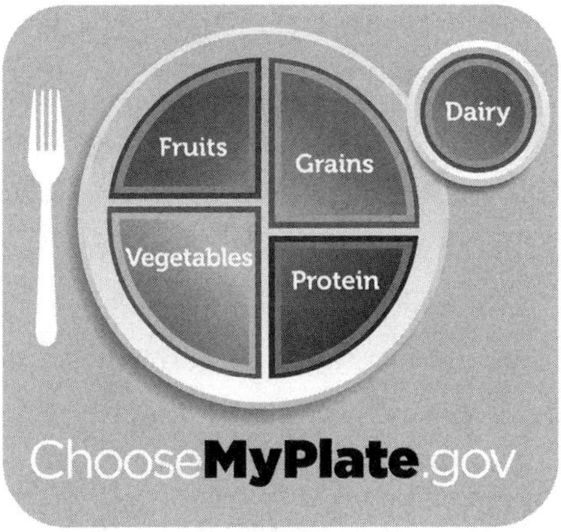

We call this the Standard American Diet or "SAD." This diet is based on reducing saturated fats and cholesterol in the diet while increasing the intake of carbohydrates, sugars, starches, and processed vegetable oils. Unfortunately, this diet negatively affects children as well as adults, because the USDA guidelines dictate what children are fed at schools. Our children (and their brains) are suffering from the calorie-restricted, low-fat, high-sugar diets they are being fed. It shouldn't be a surprise that childhood obesity has tripled since 1976.[2]

In 1997, researchers showed an inverse correlation between consuming less dietary fat and becoming obese. In other words, while fat consumption decreased 11% in the U.S. over a 20-year period, obesity increased by 32%.[3] This is hardly what the government or mainstream medical associations were expecting when we followed the food pyramid's prescriptions for healthy eating.

As previously mentioned, as a population, we have become the most obese people in history. We are suffering from a myriad of diet-related illnesses such as metabolic syndrome, diabetes, heart disease, cancer, and hypertension. Clearly, following the Standard American Diet (or SAD) program of lowering our saturated fat and cholesterol intake and relying on refined carbohydrates and processed vegetable oils has not improved our health or helped us lose weight! Instead, the opposite has occurred.

It's time for a paradigm shift in our thinking about fat and cholesterol. Fat is not the enemy! In fact, it is the preferred fuel source for the body (much better than carbohydrates, especially refined carbohydrates) and has amazing benefits for our neurological system, hormonal system, and immune system. Furthermore, our brains, nerves, tendons, ligaments, cartilage, and intestines are all made up of mostly saturated fat. We need fat to live and to thrive.

Moreover, the fat-like substance cholesterol is not the cause of heart disease; rather, cholesterol is a vital substance that is essential for life. Every cell in the body requires adequate cholesterol levels to function optimally. In fact, cholesterol is a precursor to vital hormones in the body and helps the immune system fight infections as well as acting as an anti-inflammatory agent. Keep in mind that these are just a few of the many key roles cholesterol plays in our body. We need cholesterol to live, too!

If we want to decrease our risk of heart disease, removing saturated fat and cholesterol from our diets is **not** the answer.

So, which fats should you eat and which should you avoid? This is one of the most common dietary questions that we hear from patients. First, keep in mind that not all fats are created equal. Yes, there are healthy and unhealthy dietary fats, although not the way mainstream sources would have us believe. It is important to note that the state of our health is influenced less by the **amount** of fat we eat than by the **types** of fat we eat. In Chapters 4 and 5, we will discuss which fats are good for you and which are not. We have categorized fats into the good, the bad, and the ugly to help guide you.

Because fat and cholesterol often occur together in foods, eating good fats will allow you to get proper amounts of cholesterol in your diet, too. You will learn more about why we need cholesterol in Chapter 6.

You're probably wondering if you will gain weight when you start eating additional fat. The answer can be both "yes" and "no" and is discussed further in Chapter 8. Put simply, if you eat good fats as part of a healthy diet, you will not be prone to gaining unnecessary weight. However, eating **bad** fats will increase the likelihood of weight gain because these fats cause hormonal imbalance and weight gain (as well as many other issues).

Believing that you can lose weight by eating fat will involve a mental shift in the way you view fat. The purpose of this book is to give you the real skinny on fats and to help you make the right choices about adding more good fats and oils to your diet while avoiding bad fats and oils. Doing so will put you on the right path to achieving your optimal health and weight.

## The Final Skinny:

The low-fat campaign has failed to accomplish what it set out to do. Not only has it failed to make us thinner, it has caused a rise in many chronic illnesses. It's unfortunate that the majority of doctors, medical associations, dieticians, and nutritionists continue to follow the old fat paradigm and emphasize the need to reduce fat intake by eating low- or no-fat products and substituting vegetable oils for saturated fats.

We need a complete paradigm shift about fat in order to lose those extra pounds and gain back our health and our happiness. Keep reading—in the next chapter, you'll discover some surprising "Facts about Fats" that may help you make that paradigm shift!

## (Endnotes)

1 "http://www.cdc.gov/obesity/data/facts.html. Accessed 2.13.14."

2 Prevalence of Obesity Among Children and Adolescents: United States, Trends 1963–1965 Through 2007–2008 by Cynthia Ogden, Ph.D., and Margaret Carroll, M.S.P.H., Division of Health and Nutrition Examination Surveys, "http://www.cdc.gov/nchs/data/hestat/obesity_child_07_08/obesity_child_07_08.pdf. Accessed 2.8.14".

3 Heini, Adrian, et al. Divergent Trends in Obesity and Fat Intake Patterns: The American Paradox, American Journal of Medicine. March, 1997, vol. 102:26.

# 2

# Facts About Fats

**We all grew up learning the drill:** if we just stopped eating fat, we wouldn't **be** fat. Well, it's time to unlearn that lesson, because it simply is not true. Fat is an essential part of our diet—in fact, we need fat to live!

Fat is imperative for many functions in the body, including helping us absorb minerals and fat-soluble vitamins. Fat also plays a crucial role in hormone production, maintaining healthy skin, optimizing brain function and promoting healthy organs and cells. If all of that weren't enough, fat is also the major source of energy for the body. This chapter will give you the truth about fat and why we need fat to live. These facts will make you rethink your diet and may even make you want to **increase** your fat intake. Just remember–not all fats are healthy for you. The bad fats you need to avoid are processed vegetable oils, hydrogenated oils, and trans fats. Contrary to popular belief, healthy saturated fats actually fall into the category of good fats when eaten with a balanced and varied diet.

You can use this book as your guide when choosing which fats to eat and which fats to avoid. Read on—these facts about fats might surprise you!

## *Surprising Fact #1:*
*We need fat in our diet to live!*

It's true! Every single cell in the body requires fat to function optimally. Many people, doctors included, do not understand the importance of dietary fat. The public has been led to believe that all fat in the diet must be avoided—or at least severely minimized—to avoid weight gain and heart disease. Nothing could be further from the truth. We need fat to live!

Each and every cell in the body requires fat in order to survive. We need to consume adequate levels of healthy fat from whole foods because fat provides essential nutrients for our cells as well as supporting our metabolism and hormonal production. In addition, protein cannot be adequately absorbed and utilized without the proper amounts of fat in our diets. That is why you will find fat and protein together in many of nature's foods. The most obvious example is animal meat. Furthermore, healthy fat provides a feeling of satiety, which makes us less likely to overeat. Optimal hormone production is not possible without proper amounts of fat in our diets. In addition, a healthy and balanced hormonal system is vital for having a healthy pregnancy.

Lack of fat in the diet (as well as other nutrient deficiencies) is linked to hormone disruption, infertility, and birth defects. Fat is an important component for reproduction. Did you know that when Native American couples had trouble conceiving, they went on bear fat diets? Although many women fear eating fat, good fats are not only imperative before conception, but also beneficial during pregnancy. While most of us don't have access to bear fat, another great way to get good fat is from eggs. Eggs are considered a sacred food in many cultures and are given in large quantities to pregnant women to keep them nourished. More about good fats and eggs in Chapter 4.

Bottom line: Because fat is so important to our overall health, we do not suggest eating a low-fat diet. A low-fat diet often causes numerous imbalances and mineral deficiencies and leads to insufficient amounts of fat-soluble vitamins A, D, E, and K. Furthermore, it is important to eat the right kinds of fat—i.e., good fats. Consuming the wrong types of fat can lead to poor immune systems, inadequate healing, malfunctioning hormonal systems, and weight gain.

### *Surprising Fact #2:*
*Fat DOES NOT make us fat!*

Fat has acquired a bad reputation: just open any mainstream health magazine and you'll find many articles telling us that dietary fat consumption causes weight gain and a host of medical problems. Over the last 60 years, the emphasis in the media has been on reducing fat intake. Unfortunately, we have paid attention to this message. What has happened over the last 60 years? We have markedly lowered our dietary fat intake—especially the consumption of saturated fat—through the use of low-fat and non-fat products sold in every grocery store across the United States.

The result of this anti-fat campaign is that after years of cutting back on fat, Americans are fatter than ever. Not only are we the heaviest people on the planet, we also suffer from more chronic illness than anyone else. It's obvious that anti-fat efforts haven't worked. So who has been promoting the anti-fat campaign? The list is long, but it includes mainstream medical doctors, dieticians, the American Diabetic Association, the American Heart Association, and the Academy of Nutrition and Dietetics. All of these powerful organizations (we often refer to them as The-Powers-That-Be) have convinced the public to lower their dietary fat intake. However, there is no good science to back up this advice. Simply studying biochemistry provides the correct answer about fat and leads to the conclusion that fat is a vital and essential nutrient for every cell in the body. Eliminating fat is not the answer.

Contrary to what many expect, dietary fat intake is not directly related to the amount of fat in the blood (serum levels). Rather, the amount of **carbohydrates** in the diet impacts serum levels. According to Dr. Walter Willett, chairman of the department of nutrition at the Harvard School of Public Health, fat is not the problem. "If Americans could eliminate sugary beverages, potatoes, white bread, pasta, white rice, and sugary snacks, we would wipe out almost all the problems we have with weight and diabetes and other metabolic diseases."[1]

What happens when we eat too many carbs? Carbs turn to glucose in our bodies, prompting our internal messaging systems to continue to release more and more insulin to get glucose into the cells (where it can be used as energy). Over time, the cells ultimately become more resistant to those insulin instructions—they start ignoring the annoying messenger always knocking on the door—and the pancreas needs to make more insulin to push the same amount of glucose into cells. This process results in insulin resistance.

As people become insulin resistant, carbs are a challenge for the body to process. When the pancreas gets exhausted and can't produce enough insulin to keep up with the glucose in the blood, weight gain often occurs at the same time that metabolic issues and/or diabetes develops. More about this in Chapter 7.

### *Surprising Fact #3:*
*A low-fat diet is NOT healthy!*

Over and over, we've been sternly told by The-Powers-That-Be that we must eat low-fat foods in order to be healthy. However, this is not the truth. Low-fat diets ensure that our bodies are often lacking essential nutrients such as fat-soluble vitamins, minerals, and essential fatty acids. The lack of these very important nutrients is why low-fat diets are associated with many problems, including increases in behavioral issues, childhood disease, depression, fatigue, infertility, learning disabilities, and chronic illnesses. Low-fat diets also predispose us to hormonal imbalances such as hypothyroidism. Hypothyroidism is a well-known cause of weight gain and obesity. (Please see Dr. Brownstein's book, *Overcoming Thyroid Disorders, for more information.*)

Low-fat diets have been associated with many mental, emotional, and behavioral disorders and are known to exacerbate weight gain. How does a low-fat diet lead to weight gain? The body needs and requires adequate amounts of fat to properly function. A low-fat diet will not provide sufficient fat and minerals for the body. This lack of fat and minerals will result in a stressful state in the body. The body often responds to a stressful state by slowing the metabolism down to conserve energy. Fat is then stored as the body goes into survival mode. Don't forget that low-fat diets are also often significantly higher in sugar and carbohydrates. When we eat excess sugar and carbohydrates, the body releases more insulin. Too much insulin can also lead to increased fat storage.

Another reason low-fat diets can lead to weight gain is because it's the fat in food that tells our brains we are full. Fat regulates the appetite so we don't have to eat as much. We need fat in our diets to satiate us. A low-fat diet often leaves a feeling of hunger, and that feeling can lead to overeating...and when we're hungry, we often reach for carbohydrates and grains, the so-called healthy foods the USDA promotes in its food pyramid/plate. As previously discussed, the recent changes in USDA recommendations still don't emphasize the value of healthy fat in the diet. The new food plate continues to place heavy emphasis on carbohydrates and grains as being the cornerstones of a healthy diet.

Let's look at one commonsense fact that we already all know: fat-marbled beef is corn-fed beef. Farmers have known all along that grains are what make animals fat. Farmers don't feed their cows fat to fatten them up—they feed them grains! Why? Because animals, like humans, do not feel satiety or feel full when eating grains. This means they will end up eating more because they're always hungry. The same phenomenon occurs with humans—grains make us fat. So why would the new USDA food pyramid/plate focus on increasing grain ingestion? It just does not make any sense.

"The country's big low-fat message backfired," says Dr. Frank Hu, professor of nutrition and epidemiology at the Harvard School of Public Health. "The overemphasis on reducing fat caused the consumption of carbohydrates and sugar in our diets to soar. That shift may be linked to the biggest health problems in America today."[2]

## Surprising Fact #4:

*Fat performs many essential functions in our bodies!*

Rather than something to fear or avoid, know that fat is a necessary macronutrient. Fat is important for a variety of functions in our bodies, from nutrient absorption and energy production to cell, organ, hormone, and brain function. Here's a sampling of the many vital functions of fat:

1. **Brain function.** Fat provides the structural components not only of cell membranes in the brain, but also of myelin. Myelin is the fatty insulating sheath that surrounds each nerve fiber. Proper brain function is not possible without adequate fat and myelin, the latter of which enables nerve fibers to carry messages faster.
2. **Cell membrane function.** Fat is the major constituent of the membrane that surrounds each cell of the body. If this cell membrane is disturbed or unhealthy, then the cell cannot function properly.
3. **Energy production.** Gram for gram, fat is the most efficient source of food energy. Every gram of fat provides nine calories of energy for the body versus the four calories per gram that carbohydrates and proteins provide.
4. **Hormone production.** Fat is part of the prostaglandins (or hormone-like substances) that regulate many bodily functions. These substances also regulate sex hormones.
5. **Nutrient absorption.** Fat is necessary for our intestines to absorb the fat-soluble vitamins A, D, E, and K as well as minerals. Fat-soluble vitamins are necessary ingredients for many of our bodies' physiologic and biochemical functions. Low-fat diets predispose us to mineral deficiencies.
6. **Organ protection and function.** Fat provides a cushion for our vital organs. Fat protects key organs (such as the kidneys, heart, and intestines) from injury. Fat provides the essential fatty acids necessary for many organs to function optimally.
7. **Skin health.** Healthy skin requires healthy fats, particularly essential fatty acids. Fat keeps the skin supple and smooth. Fat provides oil for the skin; in turn, the oil moisturizes the skin. Low-fat diets predispose us to dry skin conditions.

## ***Surprising Fact #5:***

*Some dietary fats are better than others!*

When it comes to fats, yes, we should play favorites. There is no question that some fats should be completely avoided. We're talking about the bad and ugly fats. The number-one fat to avoid is trans fat. Trans fat wreaks havoc on cell membranes by disrupting their normal functions. Poor cell membranes lead to a host of chronic illnesses, including diabetes, cancer, heart disease, arthritis, and fatigue. We will talk more about that later. For now, just remember that trans fat—also referred to as hydrogenated oil or partially hydrogenated oil—should be strictly avoided. This is a manufactured trans fat and definitely falls into the "ugly" fats category! More information on bad and ugly fats can be found in Chapter 5.

The good fats, however, are highly beneficial. A prime example is essential fatty acids or EFAs. EFAs are termed essential because we cannot manufacture them in our bodies and we cannot live without them. They include both omega-3 and omega-6 fats, and we need both in our bodies in proper balance. EFAs are essential for proper immune function, brain health, and cardiovascular health. They are also needed to promote healthy cell membranes.

Saturated fats are beneficial fats, too. Yes, we said **saturated** fats! These fats are necessary for utilization of the aforementioned EFAs. Furthermore, many saturated fats contain the fat-soluble vitamins A, D, E, and K, which are needed for maintaining strong and healthy cell membranes. Our bodies cannot make saturated fat out of trans fat, so if we eat too many trans fats, we will end up with the wrong fatty acids in our cell membranes. In addition, the heart, the kidneys, and muscles preferentially use saturated fats as their major source of energy. The lungs and the immune system also depend on adequate saturated fat intake to function optimally.

Saturated fats have accumulated an especially bad rap over the years from many top organizations, researchers, dieticians, doctors, and nutritionists. Don't worry—we'll talk about that in this book.

As you read further in this book in Chapters 4 and 5, you'll see that we've separated fats into three categories. There are the "good" fats that we should eat more of and the "bad" fats we should limit or even stay away from. And finally, there are also what we call the "ugly" fats. Ugly fats should be avoided at all costs!

### ***Surprising Fact #6:***
*Saturated fat is not the enemy!*

Over the last 60 years, saturated fat has been criticized by mainstream media sources, medical practitioners, dieticians and many nutritionists. Conventional wisdom tells us that almost all saturated fats are bad for us. While avoiding processed vegetable oils and trans fat is a good idea, the truth is that we actually **require** adequate amounts of saturated fat. Without it, our cells don't function properly, our hearts and brains are not properly nourished and we have hormonal imbalances and poorly functioning immune systems. In a healthy diet, saturated fat is **not** to be avoided.

Saturated fat gives our cells the strength to maintain their structure. It also plays key roles in hormonal, immune, and cardiovascular health. For example, the addition of saturated fat to the diet reduces the levels of a substance called lipoprotein (a)(Lp(a)), a substance that is strongly correlated with the risk of heart disease. Furthermore, saturated fat is required to maintain optimal brain function. Did you know that our brains are primarily made of fat? About 60%, in fact! Saturated fat is especially crucial for a baby's brain and neurological development. Learn more about fats and the brain in Chapter 9.

Foods like butter from grass-fed cows, coconut oil, and free-range eggs are all healthy sources of good fat. Bad sources of fat (the real enemies!) include processed vegetable oils, hydrogenated oils and trans fats. These are the fats that need to be avoided!

## ***Surprising Fact #7:***
## *Saturated fat and cholesterol do NOT cause heart disease!*

As previously stated, saturated fat and cholesterol do **not** cause heart disease. Let's give that a minute to sink in. But then why do so many health sources claim that saturated fat and cholesterol **do** cause heart disease?

The emphasis on reducing saturated fat and cholesterol intake started in the early 20$^{th}$ century, when a researcher fed rabbits cholesterol and the rabbits developed plaques in their aortas. These plaques were similar to the plaques humans develop. The researcher concluded that dietary cholesterol therefore caused fatty buildup in the arteries. However, the research was flawed—the rabbits were not given cholesterol in the form of natural foods, they were given pure crystalline cholesterol that had been dissolved in vegetable oil. So it's not accurate to say cholesterol in the diet causes heart disease. Furthermore, the rabbits did **not** develop the same kind of heart disease that humans do. More about this research can be found in Dr. Brownstein's book, *Drugs That Don't Work and Natural Therapies That Do.*

The theory that dietary fat raises cholesterol levels and causes heart disease gained momentum in the 1950s when a prominent medical researcher, Ancel Keys, published his Six Countries Study (and later, the more famous Seven Countries Study). Dr. Keys concluded that there was a direct relationship between the amount of saturated fat and cholesterol in the diet and the incidence of mortality from coronary heart disease. He recommended that Americans adopt a low-fat and low-cholesterol diet in order to prevent and treat heart disease.

Dr. Keys' research still reverberates today as nearly all mainstream doctors and medical organizations falsely believe that a low-fat (and low-cholesterol) diet is a heart-healthy diet. In fact, the American Heart Association and the other Powers-That-Be still recommend limiting dietary fat and cholesterol in order to prevent and treat heart disease. However, there is no good research to support these conclusions—not even Keys' own research backs up his conclusions. For example, Keys cherry-picked the data to show that a linear correlation between dietary fat and mortality from heart disease existed. How did he do that? By ignoring the majority of the data he obtained—originally, he studied 22 countries, not six or seven. When looking at the data from all 22 countries, in the majority of cases, there was no obvious correlation between the amount of dietary fat and the development of cardiovascular disease. Instead, he focused on the six (and then seven) countries that did fit his assumptions.

Keys' research and the low-fat-is-good-health dogma that came from it has led mainstream medical doctors and dieticians down the wrong road. A highly publicized report in the American Journal of Clinical Nutrition that analyzed the findings of 21 studies that followed 350,000 people for up to 23 years found **no** significant evidence correlating saturated fat intake and heart disease risk.[3] Furthermore, not only does high cholesterol not cause heart disease, it has been shown to **decrease** mortality rates, especially for the elderly.[4]

Heart disease is still the number-one killer in the U.S. After Dr. Keys' study, The-Powers-That-Be recommended that Americans lower their intake of saturated fat (from sources such as butter, coconut oil, eggs, and red meat). Furthermore, they suggested that we eat more polyunsaturated fats.

What did Americans do with that advice? They lowered the amount of saturated fat in their diets and increased their intake of polyunsaturated fats in the form of vegetable oil. Unfortunately, this change has been a disaster and, to this day, we are still suffering from the fallout of Dr. Keys' research. Since the 1950s, the mainstream health establishment and the edible oils industry have latched onto Keys' findings and promoted the use of vegetable oils such as soy, corn, and canola oils. Likewise, conventional medical sources continue to recommend lowered or zero consumption of saturated fats and cholesterol. But to this date, there are no solid studies that show that limiting saturated fat or cholesterol has any positive benefit in relation to heart disease.

We contend that switching from saturated fats to refined polyunsaturated vegetable oils has contributed—and continues to contribute—to our current epidemics of obesity, heart disease, and chronic illnesses. Along with increased rates of sugar and processed carbohydrate consumption, the Standard American Diet has become a recipe for disaster. We would be better off tossing out those "heart-healthy" processed vegetable oils and eating real food like butter and eggs again!

### ***Surprising Fact #8:***
### *Dietary fat is not the culprit of disease!*

Dietary fat has been pegged by The-Powers-That-Be as the main cause of the epidemic of chronic disease and obesity we are facing. This could not be more wrong. What **is** true is that there are plenty of dietary factors that are partly responsible for the decline of our overall health and the increase in our obesity levels. These other factors include refined foods such as processed grains (i.e., white flour), sugars (i.e., high-fructose corn syrup), and oils (i.e., corn, canola, soy) along with partially hydrogenated vegetable oils (i.e., trans fat).

Let's focus on the sugar factor first. Refined sugar—especially in the amounts consumed by the average American—can lead to diabetes, obesity, heart disease, cancer and other chronic illnesses. The consumption of refined sugar has been on the rise for the last 100 years. A century ago, we ate about a pound a year; now, we eat over 150 pounds per year! This comes in the form of candy, cookies and cakes as well as juice and soda. Just one 12-ounce soda can have eight teaspoons or more of sugar.

While unrefined sugars contain nutrients such as B-complex vitamins, chromium, and manganese, refined sugars contain no nutrients. Unfortunately for Americans, when we eat sugar, we almost always eat refined sugar—it's in everything from cereal and bread to candy and pastries. Eating this type of sugar **depletes** the body's nutrient reserves, especially the B-complex vitamins. Many diseases such as attention deficit disorder, arteriosclerosis, cancer, dental caries, diabetes, candidiasis, kidney disease, liver disease, and osteoporosis have been linked to the rise in refined sugar consumption.

Mainstream health sources have historically blamed the increase in chronic illness to the ingestion of fats, particularly saturated fats. However, as previously mentioned, fat consumption—especially the consumption of saturated fat—has **decreased** over the last 60 years. We believe a more plausible explanation for the increase in chronic illness is the increase in ingestion of refined foods such as refined sugar, refined oils, refined salt and other heavily processed foods.[5]

### *Surprising Fact #9:*

*Canola oil and other refined vegetable oils are NOT healthy for you!*

Refined vegetable oils are everywhere! We are told they are good for us, much better than saturated fat. Many people have given up on butter and replaced it with refined canola oil, soy oil, corn oil or other vegetable oils, spreads, or combinations of these bad fats. What they don't realize is that these oils are highly processed and refined and can lead to inflammation. If that weren't enough, canola, soy, and corn oils are derived from mostly genetically modified crops.

The processing of vegetable oils involves the application of very high temperatures and concentrated industrial processing methods. What's wrong with this? Well, when vegetable oils are exposed to heat and oxygen, they become rancid. Rancid oils are characterized by toxic free radicals that can damage tissues, cells and arteries. At the risk of sounding a little technical, a free radical is a molecule that has lost an electron in its outer ring. That leaves the molecule with an unpaired electron. This lone electron creates a highly unstable molecule because a substance that lacks an electron will try to steal electrons from other molecules in an effort to balance itself. This behavior quickly sets off a destructive chain reaction. When this happens, the normal functioning of cells is disrupted and inflammation is stimulated.

The more free radicals we have in our bodies, the more quickly our cells can degenerate, meaning that premature aging ensues. Furthermore, free radical damage contributes to an increased risk for many chronic illnesses, including cancer and heart disease. Until the early 1980s, restaurants and fast-food establishments used saturated sources of fat (lard or beef tallow as well as coconut and palm oils) for sautéing and deep frying. Unfortunately, now restaurants almost exclusively use polyunsaturated oils for cooking and deep frying. These oils do not hold up well to high temperatures and quickly turn rancid when used for frying and sautéing. More about cooking with fats/oils in Chapter 11.

Another issue with processed vegetable oils is the ratio of omega-3 to omega-6 essential fatty acids. A proper balance of these EFAs is needed in the body (as we will discuss further in Chapter 4). Vegetable oils are extremely high in omega-6 fatty acids and can be very inflammatory to the body. Processed vegetable oils are not healthy sources of fat. Contrary to what we have been told, these oils should be avoided or severely limited if we want to enjoy optimal health...and weight!

### *Surprising Fact #10:*
*Low-cholesterol food does NOT do your body good!*

Cholesterol and fat often occur together in nature. That's because cholesterol and fat are integral to life. Yet dietary cholesterol, like fat, has been demonized as being a cause of heart disease. Again, nothing could be further from the truth: dietary cholesterol does **not** actually have much of an impact on blood cholesterol levels. Nor does high cholesterol correlate with an increase in heart disease. More about this in Chapter 6.

Although we've been told to avoid eating cholesterol for decades, cholesterol actually plays many important roles in the body. Each cell in the body depends on adequate cholesterol in order to maintain membrane strength and stability. Furthermore, cholesterol is a precursor to hormone production—all steroid hormones are produced from cholesterol. Cholesterol is so vital that every cell in the body produces it.

Cholesterol has other essential roles in the body. It is a healing molecule that aids injury repair, and it is protective against toxic substances such as heavy metals and pesticides. Without adequate amounts of cholesterol, hormone production will not occur and the immune system will not function optimally.

Over the last 60 years, the message from The-Powers-That-Be, including Big Pharma, is clear: we need to lower our cholesterol levels to the lowest number possible. Of course, these numbers are only possible to obtain with the use of medications that interfere with the body's ability to produce cholesterol. These medications are known as statin medications. Statin drugs are the most profitable drugs in the history of Big Pharma. Statin drugs lower cholesterol by poisoning an enzyme in the body (HMG-CoA reductase). More details about statin drugs can be found in Chapter 6.

What we don't hear from the medical establishment and Big Pharma is that low cholesterol levels of less than 160mg/dl are associated with an increased risk of many illnesses, including:

- Alzheimer's disease
- Anxiety
- Cancer
- Death from any cause
- Declining brain function
- Depression
- Strokes

According to the results of a forty-year study done in Framingham, Massachusetts (The Framingham Study), the director of the study stated that "In Framingham [Massachusetts], the more saturated fat one ate, the more cholesterol one ate, the more calories one ate, the lower the person's serum [blood] cholesterol [was]. We found that the people who ate the most cholesterol, ate the most saturated fat, [and] ate the most calories weighed the least and were the most physically active." Now, that is a message Big Pharma does not want you to hear!

## SUMMARY OF SUPRISING FACTS ABOUT FATS:

*#1: We need fat in our diet to live!*

*#2: Fat DOES NOT make us fat!*

*#3: A low-fat diet is NOT healthy!*

*#4: Fat performs many essential functions in our bodies!*

*#5: Some dietary fats are better than others!*

*#6: Saturated fat is NOT the enemy!*

*#7: Saturated fat and cholesterol do NOT cause heart disease!*

*#8: Dietary fat is NOT the culprit of disease!*

*#9: Canola oil and other refined vegetable oils are NOT healthy for you!*

*#10: Low-cholesterol food does NOT do your body good!*

## (Endnotes)

1 "http://www.latimes.com/health/la-he-carbs-20101220,0,5464425.story#axzz2t0vNxYoA. Accessed 1-21-14."

2 Marni Jameson, A Reversal on Carbs, Los Angeles Times, 2010 http://www.latimes.com/health/la-he-carbs-20101220,0,5464425.story?page=1.

3 Siri-Tarino P.W., Sun Q., Hu F.B., Krauss R.M.. Meta-analysis of prospective cohort studies evaluating the association of saturated fat with cardiovascular disease, *Am J Clin Nutr.*, 2010;91:535–46.

4 Krumholz H.M. and others, *JAMA* 272, 1335–40, 1994.

5 "http://drhyman.com/blog/2014/02/07/eggs-dont-cause-heart-attacks-sugar/. Accessed 2-21-14."

# 3

# Got Fat?

**Do you eat enough fat?** Probably not—most people do not eat enough fat because they have a fear about consuming dietary fat. However, we already know from Chapter 2 that fat is **not** the enemy. It is **not** the cause of heart disease. In fact, we need fat to live! Our health is impacted by the **types** of fat we eat much more than how **much** fat we eat.

For decades, The-Powers-That-Be have claimed that unsaturated fats are "good" fats while saturated fats are "bad" fats. On the American Heart Association website, for example, saturated fat is listed as a "bad" fat while polyunsaturated fat is listed as a "better" fat.[1] Furthermore, according to Jeannie Gazzaniga-Moloo, PhD, RD, a spokeswoman for the American Dietetic Association, "Replacing saturated fats with unsaturated fats is still one of the healthiest changes most Americans can make."[2] However, the American Heart Association and The American Dietetic Association could not be more wrong. Unsaturated fats are not necessarily the healthiest fats for our bodies, especially when you consider the damaging high-temperature, industrial processing methods used to create these oils.

We will show you what fats you need to incorporate into your diet: healthy saturated, monounsaturated, and some polyunsaturated, plus which fats you should minimize, such as refined or hydrogenated fats and processed polyunsaturated fats. We'll give you examples of which fats are prevalent in various food sources. Finally, we will discuss how the refining process affects fats and oils. But before we get into good fats and bad fats, you need to understand some basic properties of fats.

## What is Fat?

Despite decades of confusion and misunderstanding surrounding fat, its basic properties aren't too complicated. Fat, along with proteins and carbohydrates, is an important source of energy for the human body. These three substances are collectively known as dietary macronutrients.

Fat is made up of complex chemical compounds called fatty acids. (For the chemistry majors who are reading this, a fatty acid contains a carboxylic acid with a long aliphatic tail.) The types of fatty acids that are present in the fat determine if the fat is saturated or unsaturated. In the simplest terms, fatty acids without double bonds are called saturated. Fatty acids with double bonds are called unsaturated. A fat molecule is monounsaturated if it contains one double bond and polyunsaturated if it contains more than one double bond.

But perhaps the most basic and easy-to-understand aspect of fat is that it is the best dietary source of energy: fat contains nine calories per gram, whereas proteins and carbohydrates only offer four calories per gram.

## What is the Difference Between a Fat and an Oil?

From a technical point of view, a fat can be either solid or liquid at room temperature. In conversational terms, if a fat is solid at room temperature (as is the case with saturated fat), it's called a fat. A good example of a fat is butter. However, if a fat is liquid at room temperature (as is the case with unsaturated fat), it is considered to be an oil. A good example of an oil is olive oil.

## How Are Fats Categorized?

There are two major categories of fats: saturated and unsaturated. Unsaturated includes both monounsaturated and polyunsaturated fats (such as those found in nuts, vegetable oils, and fish). While we will discuss these categories in detail later in this chapter, for now you need to know that these terms refer to the chemical structure of fats. In Figure 3, you can see the different chemical structures of unsaturated and saturated fatty acids.

Each of these types of fat is defined by the number of carbon and hydrogen atoms that are present in the fat's chemical structure. That chemical structure of the fatty acid dictates the stability of the fat. Saturated fats are "saturated" with hydrogen atoms and have no double bonds or bends in their structure. This makes them very stable fats even when heated to high temperatures.

Unsaturated fats are not as stable at high temperatures because they contain double bonds which can be hydrogenated. The double bonds provide flexibility and bends in the chemical structure which can make it unstable when heated. That means unsaturated fats can oxidize and become rancid very easily when exposed to heat, oxygen and/or light.

**FIGURE 3: Saturated VS Unsaturated Fatty Acids**

Saturated Fatty Acid

Unsaturated Fatty Acid

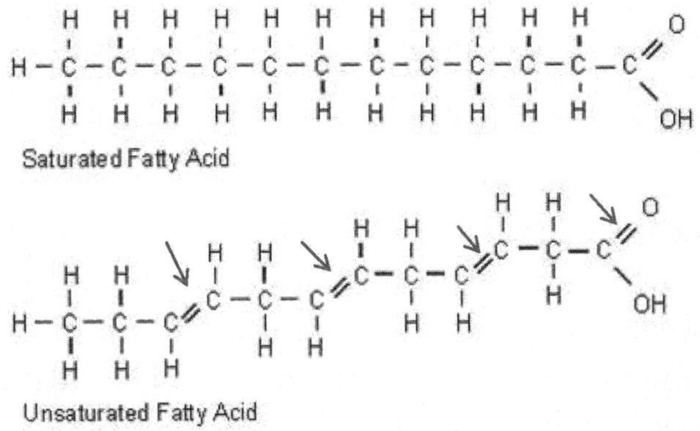

Figure 3: Example of saturated versus unsaturated fatty acids. The double bonds in the unsaturated fatty acid are delineated by the arrows. Saturated fats do not contain any double bonds.

But guess what? No fat is 100% saturated or unsaturated. In nature, fats are made up of a mixture of various fatty acids. Many people think that pork lard is a saturated fat. Not true! It actually contains 41% saturated fat, 47% monounsaturated fat and 11% polyunsaturated fat. On the flip side, although olive oil is thought of as a strictly monounsaturated fat, it's actually comprised of 75% monounsaturated fat, 14% saturated fat, and 11% polyunsaturated fat.

Put simply, different foods have different mixtures of fatty acids. Nature intended it that way since there are no totally "bad" or "good" fatty acids. A healthy diet includes a balanced concentration of all fats: polyunsaturated, monounsaturated...and yes, saturated fats, too!

## What Are Saturated Fats?

As previously stated, if a fat is saturated, that means that all of that fat's carbon atoms are bonded to hydrogen atoms and the chemical structure contains no double bonds. Figure 4 shows an example of a saturated fatty acid.

**FIGURE 4: Saturated Fatty Acid**

```
  H H H H H H H H H H H H H H H H H
  | | | | | | | | | | | | | | | | |  O
H-C-C-C-C-C-C-C-C-C-C-C-C-C-C-C-C-C-C⁼
  | | | | | | | | | | | | | | | | |  \
  H H H H H H H H H H H H H H H H H   OH
```

Because saturated fats have no double bonds and are fully saturated with hydrogen atoms, saturated fats have a straight structure with no kinks or bends. The saturated carbon bonds provide a very stable structure. That's why saturated fats can withstand cooking at higher temperatures yet maintain their structure.

In other words, when saturated fats are heated, they don't produce tissue-damaging free radicals the way unsaturated fats can. Plus, saturated fats don't go rancid or oxidize when exposed to light, oxygen and/or heat. This stability makes saturated fats safer to store for longer lengths of time.

## What Are Sources of Saturated Fats?

Remember, saturated fats are solid or firm at room temperature. Tropical oils (coconut and palm oil) and animal food sources (meat, dairy, eggs) contain large amounts of saturated fats. Saturated fats from healthy food sources provide important nutrition for the body! The most nutritious foods include grass-fed/free-range animal products and coconut oil. Different sources of saturated fats are listed in Table 1.

**Table 1: Foods That Contain Significant Amounts of Saturated Fats**

| | |
|---|---|
| Butter | Eggs |
| Cheese | Ghee (clarified butter) |
| Coconut Cream/Milk | Meat |
| Coconut Oil | Palm Oil |
| Dairy Milk and Cream | Tallow |

## What Are Monounsaturated Fats?

Monounsaturated fats are liquid or soft at room temperature and firm at cooler temperatures. If they are not highly processed, monounsaturated fats contain vitamin E. However, high heat can disrupt this antioxidant vitamin. Monounsaturated fats are missing two hydrogen atoms—their structure contains one double bond between two carbon atoms. Figure 5 shows the chemical structure of a monounsaturated fatty acid.

**FIGURE 5: Monounsaturated Fatty Acid**

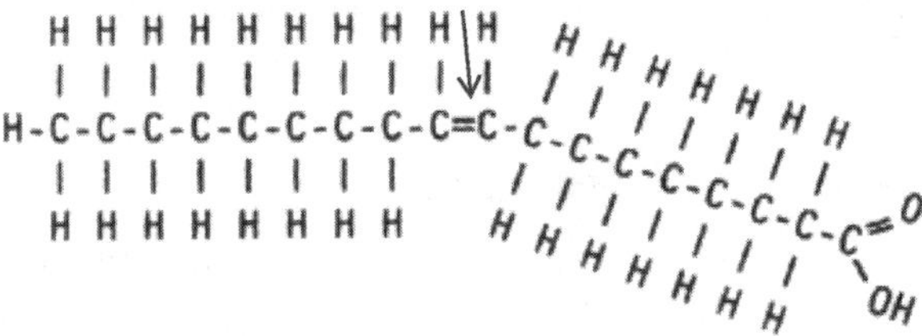

Figure 5: Example of Monounsaturated Fat. Note the double bond is delineated with an arrow.

The double bond makes monounsaturated fats less stable than saturated fats and therefore less suitable for high-heat cooking.

Technicalities aside, what you really need to know is this: don't use monounsaturated fats for high-heat cooking. Instead, use them for low- to medium-heat cooking and in no-heat situations, like dressing salads, tossing with cooked whole grains, and in dips like hummus. Or garnish an already-cooked dish with monounsaturated fats. Table 2 lists some sources of monounsaturated fats.

## What are Sources of Monounsaturated Fats?

The most common form of monounsaturated fat is oleic acid, which is high in olive oil. Other common forms are almonds, and avocado as well as those items listed below in Table 2. Remember, all fats are a blend of monounsaturated, polyunsaturated, and saturated fats.

**Table 2: Sources of Monounsaturated Fats**

| | |
|---|---|
| Almonds | Olive Oil |
| Avocado | Peanuts |
| Avocado Oil | Pecans |
| Canola Oil* | Pistachios |
| Cashews | Sesame Oil (cold pressed) |
| Duck Fat | Salad Dressings (homemade) |
| Hazelnuts | Schmaltz (chicken/goose fat) |
| Lard | Skin on Poultry |
| Macadamias | Spreads* |

* *Listed as a source of monounsaturated oils, but not one we recommend*

## What are Polyunsaturated Fats?

Polyunsaturated fats are liquid at room temperature. Structurally speaking, polyunsaturated fats are missing two or more hydrogen pairs and have two or more double bonds between carbon atoms in their chemical structure. The most common forms of polyunsaturated fats in our diets are the essential fatty acids (EFAs) that are known as omega-3 and omega-6 fatty acids. The "-3" and "-6" refer to a specific location of the first double bond. Figure 6 and 7 are examples of the chemical structure of omega-3 and omega-6 fatty acids.

Omega-3 fatty acids are also referred to as alpha-linolenic acid (ALA). Fish oil and flax oils are examples of omega-3 fatty acids. Omega-6 fatty acids are often referred to as linoleic acid (LA). Vegetable oils such as canola, corn, safflower, and soybean are examples of oils high in omega-6 fatty acids of the short chain variety and evening primrose, borage, and black currant oil are long chain sources.

**FIGURE 6: Omega-3 Fatty Acid**

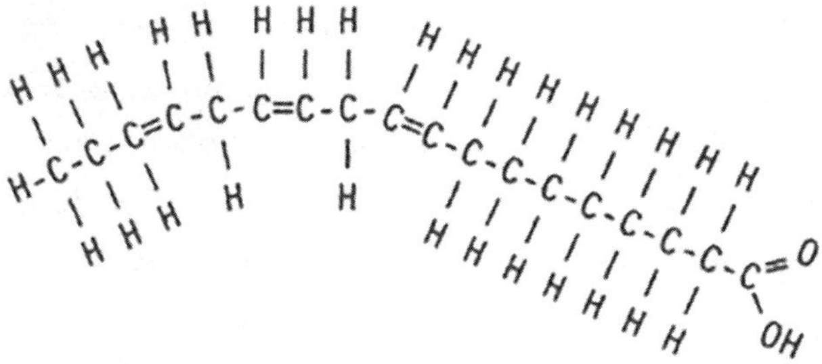

**FIGURE 7: Omega-6 Fatty Acid**

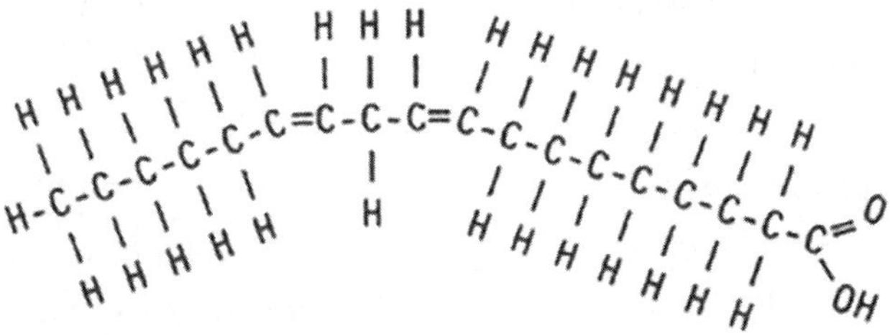

It is important to remember that because polyunsaturated fats/oils have multiple double bonds and kinks in their chemical structures, they can't pack together tightly and they are **not stable** when exposed to heat, light, and/or oxygen. Heat is able to bend and disrupt the normal structure of any fatty acid that contains double bonds. **Polyunsaturated fats are the least stable of all the fats.** Unlike saturated fats, they cannot withstand high-heat processing or high-heat cooking because the heat causes the structure of the fats to break down and become damaged and rancid. Plus, free radicals are easily formed when the chemical structure is damaged, and free radicals lead to inflammation and are associated with nearly all chronic illnesses. You want to minimize or eliminate food sources in your diet that promote free radical formation.

## What Are Free Radicals?

Free radicals are compounds that damage the cells of the body and contribute to diseases such as cancer, autoimmune disorders, diabetes, obesity, and heart disease. Although many polyunsaturated oils such as canola, grapeseed, and soybean oil are promoted as being ideal for baking and cooking purposes, these oils are not optimal in a healthy diet—they've already been damaged by heavy refining processes. Hence, nearly all supermarket oils are rancid before they even hit the store shelves. These oils should be avoided.

Healthy oils are cold-pressed or expeller-pressed. In the case of olive oil, unprocessed oil is called extra-virgin. These minimally processed oils are packaged in dark containers that shield the oils from light. When you taste an unprocessed oil, you'll find that it does not have a bitter or rancid taste (or smell).

Generally speaking, the oils to avoid are the ones that are sold in clear plastic containers. Most of these oils have been highly processed with methods that cause all of the oil's antioxidants to be removed. Also, these oils are often bleached and deodorized so that consumers won't notice their rancidity.

## What Are Sources of Polyunsaturated Fats?

Examples of polyunsaturated fats are shown in Table 3. As previously mentioned, common polyunsaturated fats include oils with high levels of omega-3 and omega-6 components. These components are also known as "essential fatty acids" or EFAs. Not all polyunsaturated fats or EFA's are healthy for you. For example, grapeseed oil is often promoted as a healthy fat to cook with when in fact it is always rancid and processed—you need hexane to leach out the tiny bit of oil the scrap seeds contain after they've been pressed to make wine, and it should be avoided. Furthermore, as previously mentioned, canola, corn, cottonseed, and soybean oils are all processed vegetable oils you should also steer clear of.

**Table 3: Sources of Polyunsaturated Oils**

| Omega-3 Fatty Acids | Omega-6 Fatty Acids |
|---|---|
| Chia Seeds | Borage |
| Cod Liver Oil | Black Currant |
| Cold Water Fish *(mackerel, salmon, albacore tuna, sardines, lake trout)* | Corn* |
| | Cottonseed* |
| | Grapeseed Oil* |
| Flaxseeds | Primrose |
| Flaxseed Oil | Safflower* |
| Pumpkin Seeds and Oil | Sesame |
| Nuts and Nut Oils *(e.g., walnuts, pecans, almonds, etc)* | Soybean* |
| | Sunflower* |

** Listed as a source of polyunsaturated oils, but not one we recommend*

## What are Essential Fatty Acids?

The polyunsaturated forms called omega-3 oil (alpha linolenic acid or ALA) and omega-6 oil (linoleic acid or LA) are called "essential" fatty acids because the body cannot manufacture them. Our lives depend on getting adequate amounts of essential fatty acids from our diets. These essential fatty acids (EFAs) play important roles in all of our cells. The brain cells, nerve endings or synapses, sense organs, adrenal glands, and sex glands all rely on EFAs. Our bodies also need EFAs to produce the hormone-like prostaglandins necessary for the regulating and communicating of cells.

While we are on the topic of omega-3s, let's explore them in more detail. Omega-3 fats in the form of ALA and omega-6 fats in the form of LA are known as short-chain EFAs. Long-chain omega-3 and omega-6 fatty acids called docosahexaenoic acid (or DHA) and eicosapentaenoic acid (or EPA) are derived from these parent short chain omega-3's ALA and LA. DHA is necessary for brain, eye, and nerve health. It is also an important factor for our immune system's inflammatory response thus making it necessary for reducing many degenerative diseases. EPA also plays a role in reducing inflammation and is a precursor to DHA.

Unfortunately, due to changes in our modern lifestyles and dietary choices (particularly due to high intake of omega-6 vegetable oils), some people cannot convert short-chain EFAs to long-chain EFAs very efficiently. That means many people are deficient in those crucial long-chain EFAs. For example, while flax seed oil is touted as being a good source of omega-3 fats, it contains only the short-chain omega-3 fatty acids. As a result, sometimes only a small percentage of the parent omega-3 fatty acid ALA consumed in the diet is converted to the more important long-chain fatty acids such as DHA, EPA, and anti-inflammatory eicosanoids. Furthermore, saturated fat is necessary in the diet in order for the body to properly utilize the omega-3's in flax oil. That means it's important to consume both plant and animal sources of omega-3 fatty acids.

If you're looking for good dietary sources of DHA and EPA, you'll find them in egg yolks from pastured hens, liver (particularly in liver from animals that are pastured/grass-fed), shellfish, as well as oily fish (such as anchovies and wild salmon). And not only is cod liver oil a source of DHA and EPA, it's also more importantly a good source of the fat-soluble vitamins A and D. Many people are deficient in these important nutrients due to eating low-fat diets. That said, not all cod liver oil is created equally! It is important to get cod liver oil that has not been highly processed. Appendix B provides a list of good sources of cod liver oil. If you opt to take any omega-3 supplements, however, remember to monitor yourself carefully or take the supplements with doctor supervision so that you do not create an imbalance with omega-6 fats in your body. Furthermore, people who consume large amounts of fatty fish, fish oil, or cod liver oil may face adverse consequences from consuming an excess of the omega-3 fatty acid eicosapentaenoic acid (EPA).[3]

## What About Fish Oil?

We do not recommend fish oil as a supplement (note: cod liver oil is not the same as fish oil). Most fish oils on the market are highly refined very similar to the way vegetable oils are refined. Refining, degumming, deodorization, etc. are just some of the processes used on fish oil. The end product is an ineffective supplement that is full of damaged, isolated omega-3's. Taking fish oil supplements may actually lead to the opposite effect you are looking for by adding omega-3's to your diet. Studies show that one gram per day of omega-3 fatty acids from fish oil reduces cardiovascular mortality in patients with chronic heart failure or those who have recently had a heart attack. However, fish oil may increase cardiovascular and total mortality, especially when used for more than four years in combination with a standard modern diet.[4] Keep in mind, nutrients in **real** food are more bioavailable than in supplements.

## What About Omega-6's in the Form of Arachidonic Acid or Gamma-Linolenic Acid?

Omega-6 fatty acids are also available either in short chain form—linoleic acid (LA)—or long chain form—arachidonic acid (AA) or gamma-linolenic acid (GLA). As previously mentioned, the LA form of omega-6 fats is overabundant in our diets in the form of vegetable oils such as corn, soybean, and safflower oils, and this overabundance can create inflammatory issues in the body. Furthermore, some conditions like alcoholism and insulin resistance decrease our ability to convert short chain LA to long chain AA.[5] AA, on the other hand, is an important part of cell membranes and also assists in blood clotting, inflammation regulation, and cell communication. This long-chain fat is found in animal foods such as egg yolks, liver, meat, and seafood. GLA helps in the production of prostaglandins, which are locally produced tissue hormones that regulate many bodily functions. GLA is an effective anti-inflammatory agent, yet very little GLA is found in the diet. Borage oil is the richest supplemental source, followed by black currant oil and evening primrose oil. Sometimes doctors may use these supplements to help with arthritis, autoimmune disorders, premenstrual syndrome and for healthy growth of skin, hair, and nails.

## What is The Proper Balance of Essential Fatty Acids?

A good balance of EFAs keeps us healthy. That balance includes both omega-6 fatty acids and omega-3 fatty acids. It appears that a ratio between 2:1 and 4:1 of omega-6 fats to omega-3 fats provides the optimal amounts of essential fatty acids for the body. Despite this, we tend to get too many poor-quality omega-6 fats in our diet since they are far more prevalent in the commercial meats, eggs, dairy, and processed foods commonly found in the Standard American Diet (SAD). For example, commercial factory-"farmed" meat contains a ratio of 25:1 of omega-6 fats to omega-3 fats, whereas free-range/pastured/wild animal products contain a 2:1 ratio of these fats. In addition, the refined vegetable oils that are used in fast foods and most snack foods (cookies, crackers, sweets) are also a major source of poor-quality omega-6 fats in the diet.

Eating the Standard American Diet can make an excess of bad omega-6 fats add up quickly in your body, and those omega-6 fats lead to inflammation. Inflammation is the root of almost every chronic illness we see today. Having an imbalance of omega-3 and omega-6 fats is linked to many health concerns including cardiovascular disease, cancer, and autoimmune diseases.[6] Other health issues from EFA imbalance are listed in Table 4. (EFAs will be discussed further in the next chapter.)

**Table 4: Health Issues From Imbalances of EFAs**

| | |
|---|---|
| Accelerated Aging | Heart Attacks |
| ADD/ADHD | Immune Dysfunction |
| Alzheimer's | Insulin Resistance |
| Arthritis | Lupus |
| Asthma | Mental Disorders |
| Cancer | Obesity |
| Depression | Poor Healing |
| Diabetes | Postpartum Depression |
| Eczema | Schizophrenia |
| Epilepsy | Stroke |
| Hair Loss | |

## What About Omega-9 Fats?

Omega-9 fats are often confused as being one of the essential fatty acids. However, omega-9 fats are **not** essential since our bodies can manufacture them. Therefore, they do not need to be consumed in the diet regularly as do omega-3 fats and omega-6 fats. Omega-9 (which is a monounsaturated fat also known as oleic acid) is found in olive oil as well as olives, avocados, almonds, peanuts, cashews, sesame, hazelnuts, and macadamia nuts.

## What Are Long- and Short-Chain Fats?

Another way fats are classified is by the length of the chain of their fatty acids. Most naturally occurring fatty acids have a chain of an even number of carbon atoms, from 4 to 28.[7] Fats are classified by their length: they are short-, medium-, long- and very-long-chain fatty acids.

**Short-chain (4–6 carbons) fatty acids** are saturated. Common examples are butyric acid (butter) and caprylic acid (coconut oil). Butyric acid feeds healthy bacteria and supports gut health, while caprylic acid inhibits the growth of yeast and candida.

**Medium-chain (8–12 carbons) fatty acids** are also commonly found in butter and coconut oil as well as in breast milk. Lauric and capric acids are used for energy as well as being highly anti-bacterial, anti-viral and anti-fungal.

**Long-chain (14–18 carbons) fatty acids** come in all three forms: saturated (stearic acid in beef), monounsaturated (oleic acid in olive oil and palmitoleic acid in animal fats) and polyunsaturated (omega-6 fats and omega-3 fats). Stearic acid is important in the diet because it is the main fat for the heart.

**Very-long-chain (20–24 carbons) fatty acids** are unsaturated and often have multiple double bonds. The most commonly known of these are eicosapentaenoic acid (EPA) and docosahexaenoic acid (DHA), which are abundant in fish and in cod liver oil and are necessary for brain and eye health.

One key benefit of both short-and medium-chain fatty acids is that they provide immune system support due to their antimicrobial properties which protect us from viruses, bacteria, parasites, and yeast. And since these fats do not need bile salts to be digested, they are quickly absorbed in the body for energy. Short- and medium-chain fats also stimulate the metabolism. In fact, these saturated fats can aid with weight loss. This is one reason coconut oil is now being touted as a good fat for weight loss. In other words, eating **more** of this fat actually helps you **lose** weight! More about fat and weight loss in Chapter 8.

## What Are Trans-Fats

Trans-fats are formed through a chemical process called hydrogenation. This process begins with an unsaturated fat, which lacks hydrogen atoms and has at least one double bond (remember, that structure makes unsaturated fats unstable). Hydrogenation is a chemical process achieved with the presence of a catalyst like platinum or nickel that forces an unsaturated fatty acid to accept additional hydrogen atoms into their bonds, making them, in effect, partially saturated or partially hydrogenated. These are also called trans fats. Margarine is the most common example of a hydrogenated trans fat. Trans fats are present in all foods that have been hydrogenated or partially hydrogenated.

Why is this done? Hydrogenation increases the shelf life of foods, which leads to greater profits for food manufacturers since the odorless, colorless, flavorless refined oils that result from the hydrogenation process do not have an expiration date. The only benefit of hydrogenation is increasing the manufacturer's bottom line.

Margarine, shortening, and any food that lists "hydrogenated oil" or "partially hydrogenated oil" in its ingredient list contains trans fats. Trans fats are toxic substances for our cell membranes. When our cells contain an overabundance of trans fats, the cells become leaky and distorted; in effect, they themselves become partially hydrogenated. This can promote vitamin and mineral deficiencies. The consumption of partially hydrogenated vegetable oils and the trans fats that are formed during this process has been linked to increases in cancer, heart disease and many other chronic degenerative disorders. Trans fats are truly the "ugly" fats.

We discuss trans fats and hydrogenation further in Chapter 5. For now, all you need to remember is that we suggest you completely avoid any food that contains trans fats.

## The Final Skinny:

Fat can be classified in many different ways. The key to remember is that **we need a variety of fats and oils in our diets**. A healthy diet includes a combination of saturated, monounsaturated, and polyunsaturated fats and oils. But also remember that not all types of fats and oils are healthy for you. In the following chapters, we have divided the fats into categories: the good, the bad, and the ugly. That way, you can focus on including more good fats in your diet. There is no question that we need more of these good fats to achieve and maintain optimal health. And don't forget to avoid food with those ugly trans fats!

# (Endnotes)

1 From www.heart.org, Accessed 1.28.14.
2 "http://www.webmd.com/diet/healthy-kitchen-11/omega-fatty-acids, Accessed 1.12.14".
3 "http://www.westonaprice.org/know-your-fats/precious-yet-perilous, Accessed 2.12.14".
4 "http://www.westonaprice.org/know-your-fats/precious-yet-perilous, Accessed 2.12.14".
5 Nakamura M.T., Nara T.Y.. Structure, function, and dietary regulation of delta6, delta5, and delta9 desaturases, *Annu Rev Nutr.* 2004;24:345–376.
6 Biomed Pharmacother., 2002 Oct;56(8):365–79.
7 *IUPAC Compendium of Chemical Terminology* (2nd ed.), International Union of Pure and Applied Chemistry, 1997, ISBN 0-521-51150-X. Retrieved 2007-10-31.

# 4

# Fat: The Good

**Rather than being something to fear or avoid** or feel guilty about eating, fat is a vital and necessary ingredient in our diets. Fat plays many important roles in the body, including creating healthy cells and supplying the body with essential ingredients necessary for proper immune system and hormonal functioning. Dietary fat also helps maintain healthy skin, hair, and eyes.

However, not all fats are healthy for you: there are good, bad, and ugly fats. This chapter will educate you about the good fats and how to incorporate them into your diet. Good fats are those that have not been hydrogenated, manufactured with high heat or otherwise damaged in processing.

This chapter will explain why good fats are not dietary enemies. We will get to the real dietary enemies–the bad and the ugly fats—in the next chapter. For now, let's focus on the good fats. We suggest you go out of your way to enjoy these fats regularly.

## What Are The "Good" Fats?

It's a simple definition: good fats have not been hydrogenated, refined, over-processed with high heat, bleached, deodorized, or damaged at home due to improper storage or cooking methods. Good fats are used by the body to maintain cellular architecture and are also used to produce energy. Every cell requires the presence of good fats. Furthermore, our bodies use good fats to maintain healthy immune and hormonal systems. Luckily, good fats come in many different forms.

## Where Are Good Fats Found?

Good fats can be found in both saturated and unsaturated fats. Remember, in nature, all fats are a combination of monounsaturated, polyunsaturated, and saturated fats. Good fats that are saturated are found in butter, ghee (which is clarified butter), coconut oil, palm oil, and tallow. They are also found in animal foods such as pastured eggs, dairy, and meat. Good fats that are monounsaturated are found in extra-virgin olive oil, lard, schmaltz (that's chicken or goose fat) or unrefined sesame and avocado oils and whole avocados. Finally, good fats in the form of mostly polyunsaturated fats are found in fish, chia seeds, flaxseeds, walnuts or other nuts and seeds and their oils, as well as black currant seed and evening primrose oils.

See Table 5 for an outline of the good fats that should be included in a healthy diet. Keep in mind the highest quality oils are packaged in dark, opaque containers and are cold-pressed, expeller-pressed, or—in the case of olive oil—extra-virgin.

**Table 5: List of Good Fats**

**Saturated:**
Butter, coconut oil, ghee (clarified butter), palm oil, tallow, and animal foods including pastured eggs, dairy, and meat.

**Monounsaturated:**
Olive oil, lard, avocado, expeller-pressed sesame oil, chicken/duck/goose fat

**Polyunsaturated (omega-3 fats and omega-6 fats, a.k.a. Essential Fatty Acids or EFAs):**
Chia seeds, cod liver oil, flax oil and seeds, fish, walnuts and other nuts/seeds and their oils, black currant seed oil, evening primrose oil

## Is Saturated Fat Unhealthy?

Many of us have been led to believe that saturated fat is a bad fat and should be avoided like the plague. And who could blame us for thinking this way? For over 60 years, The-Powers-That-Be have inappropriately demonized saturated fat. It's time to set the record straight!

Saturated fatty acids are necessary for many important functions in the body and are part of a healthy diet. Our cells need saturated fat for strength and integrity, plus saturated fat provides a great source of energy and makes us feel satiated after a meal. Saturated fat is needed for cardiovascular, liver, and bone health, as well as proper functioning of our brains, lungs, nerves, tendons, ligaments, cartilage, and intestines. Stearic acid, a saturated fat, is the main food for the heart.

In short, saturated fats are needed for almost every system in our body to function optimally. In particular, the medium-chain saturated fatty acids such as lauric and capric acids have been found to play an important role in supporting the immune system. These medium-chain saturated fats have potent antibacterial and antiviral properties.

## But, What Exactly Is Good About Saturated Fat?

Many vital nutrients and substances are only found in saturated fat, and many other vital nutrients can only be of use to our bodies if they're eaten along with fat. The fat-soluble vitamins A, D, E, and K, for instance, are essential nutrients in our diet because we cannot manufacture the majority of them in our bodies. The exception is vitamin D, which can be manufactured in the skin with the help of sufficiently strong sunlight.

In order to maintain optimal levels of fat-soluble essential vitamins in our bodies, we need fat in our diets, especially saturated fat. Optimal forms of saturated fat are only found in animal foods. Due to brainwashing from The-Powers-That-Be, we have decreased our consumption of animal foods over the years (we don't eat nearly as much grass-fed meats and organ meats, grass-fed butter, pastured eggs, and grass-fed dairy products as we used to) and are consequently missing out on these important essential vitamins. The following is a list of just some of the many benefits of the fat-soluble vitamins A, D, E, and K:

**Vitamin A**—Improves and maintains vision, essential for maintenance and optimal functioning of the cornea, epithelial cells, soft tissue, mucus membranes, skin, bone and tooth growth, reproduction, immunity.

**Vitamin D**—Necessary for proper functioning of the organ systems, regulates calcium and phosphate levels, promotes bone formation and immune system functioning.

**Vitamin E**—Has antioxidant capabilities and supports red blood cell function as well as aiding in skin healing and scar reduction.

**Vitamin K**—Necessary for blood clotting, regulates bone metabolism, prevents calcification of organs and soft tissues and regulates blood sugar.

Please note: there are multiple forms of Vitamin K, with the most common being K1 and K2. While K1 is mostly associated with blood clotting in the body, K2 is being researched more and more. Researchers are finding that K2 is needed to make sure calcium ends up where it needs to be—namely, in our bones and teeth rather than our tissues.

This critical form of vitamin K is only found in animal foods, particularly egg yolks, cheese, and butter (if organic). When cows have been eating rapidly growing green grass, the levels of K2 in their milk and meat is higher. Butter oil with high levels of K2 is a great source of this important nutrient and has been shown to have a synergistic effect with cod liver oil in the body. More information and sources of high-vitamin butter oil can be found at: www.greenpasture.org.

Vitamin K2 is necessary for utilization of calcium and Vitamin D in the body, and it is needed for calcium to be mineralized into bone. Vitamin K2 has been shown to improve diabetes, heart disease, various cancers, bone and dental health, kidney disease, Alzheimer's, brain and nerve health, aging and wrinkles, varicose veins, and arthritis. K2 is also critical for fertility, pregnancy, and prenatal development.

Research shows that vitamins A, D, and K2 interact and work synergistically in the body along with other minerals (e.g., calcium, zinc, and magnesium).[1]

## Are All Saturated Fats Healthy For You?

There are some saturated fats we suggest you avoid. These are the saturated fats found in animal products sourced from animals that are from feedlots (also called factory-farmed animals). The official term for these industrial animal processing centers is a "Centralized Animal Feeding Operation" or CAFO. Most of the meat in America comes from CAFOs. Animals raised under these unsanitary conditions are under continual stress and are constantly sick. They are raised in crowded dirt lots or in factory-sized buildings and packed together by the thousands. Frequently, they are forced to stand day in and day out on concrete floors often never breathing fresh air, seeing daylight or walking outside. They must stand, sit, and lay in their own excrement due to overcrowding.

Moreover, they're usually kept in artificial lighting conditions, sometimes in constant dark and sometimes in constant light. The latter is the case with hens since the constant light forces them to overproduce eggs. Most of these animals are fed genetically modified grains, chicken litter (that's chicken droppings, chicken feathers and discarded bits of chicken) and other byproducts of animal processing. They also regularly receive antibiotics, hormones, and bakery waste scraps that often contain trans fat.

Despite the idyllic paintings of cows in the field that often accompany the packaging of products made from these animals, they are not out on the pasture eating healthy green grass and insects the way they're meant to. Instead, they're kept in CAFOs where they become very sick and disease-laden. That's why they're given so many antibiotics and hormones—without those drugs, the animals would die.

Since fat tissues are where animals store toxins, the fat from these animals contains pesticides, herbicides, stress hormones, growth hormones, and antibiotics, all of which are then passed along to us when we eat food made with these highly processed animal products. Unfortunately, unless animal products say they're grass-fed/pastured, the majority of products sold in supermarkets, restaurants and even health food stores has been sourced from CAFOs.

Avoiding fast food, processed food and cheap food will help you avoid these unhealthier forms of saturated fat. But CAFO meat is not to be confused with grass-fed meat from healthy pastured animals. We **do** recommend eating animal products from organic and grass-fed/pastured/

free-range, hormone-free, antibiotic-free, healthy animals, because those products are good sources of healthy saturated fats (and other healthful nutrients, too!).

It's also worth noting that simply buying meat that is organic does not mean it's healthy for you. The animals need to be grass-fed and not grain-fed in order for us to obtain the proper nutrients and health-enhancing benefits of meat.

## What Is the Difference Between Grass-Fed and Grain-Fed Meat?

Cows were meant to get their nutrients from eating grass. Grass-fed beef is full of healthy nutrients, including essential fatty acids for the brain and body as well as conjugated linoleic acid (CLA), which has anti-cancer and anti-infective properties. Read on for more benefits of grass-fed meat from www.grasslandbeef.com Find grass-fed, pastured meats near you at www.localharvest.com or www.eatwild.com.

**Grass-fed meat has wonderful qualities:**

- Four times more CLA than grain-fed beef (CLA benefits include: anti-carcinogenic, increases lean body mass, prevents arteriosclerosis, slows or halts diabetes)
- High in branch-chain amino acids
- Ideal ratio of omega-6 fats to omega-3 fats (a 3:1 ratio, which is similar to the ratio found in fish)
- No animal byproducts
- No hormones
- No irradiation
- No antibiotics
- One-third fewer calories than grain-fed beef
- Risk of E. coli bacteria is minimal
- Three to six times more vitamin A and vitamin E than grain-fed beef; both of these nutrients reduce the risk of cancer and heart disease

**vs.**

**Grain-fed beef has not-so-wonderful qualities:**

- Antibiotics added daily to feed ration
- Greater risk of E. coli bacteria due to grain diet causing acidic digestive system
- Growth-stimulating hormone routinely used
- Insignificant amount of CLA
- Less than 25% of the vitamins A and E of grass-fed beef
- More total fat (with a poor omega-6 fat to omega-3 fat ratio)
- Thirty percent more calories than grass-fed beef

## What About USDA Prime Meats?

Many people think the label "USDA Prime" on meat means that it is healthier. What that label actually means is that there is a certain amount of marbling (or fat streaks) in the beef. However, in order to develop the complex marbling required to be graded "Prime," cattle need to be fed a lot of corn. Cattle fed a lot of corn also need copious amounts of antibiotics to stay alive since corn is not the proper food for cattle—it makes them sick. Then why do it? Feeding corn to cattle can fatten them quickly, and the faster the manufacturer can fatten cattle for slaughter, the faster the manufacturer will make more money, plus they can sell meat labeled USDA Prime for a higher price.

Look for beef from grass-fed cattle. Cattle were designed to eat grass, and they pass on healthy nutrients to us. Furthermore, grass-fed cattle live less stressed lives, are better for the environment and support sustainable farming.

## Are Animal Fats Really Healthy For You?

According to research done by Dr. Weston A. Price (www.westonaprice.org), all people living in traditional cultures consumed some sort of animal foods. The most prized parts were the organ meats and fat. The animal foods and fat came from a variety of sources: eggs, milk, fish, seafood, water and land fowl, animals, and even insects. While conducting his research, Dr. Price found that compared to the Standard American Diet, traditional animal-based diets contained at least four times the levels of calcium and other minerals and ten times the level of fat-soluble vitamins. In our practice, we find that many patients who avoid animal fats are deficient in fat-soluble vitamins A, D, E, and K as well as minerals.

Animal fats contain many nutrients that protect against cancer and heart disease. Conversely, elevated rates of cancer and heart disease are associated with consumption of large amounts of polyunsaturated fats in the form of vegetable oils.[2]

Despite the crucial benefits that animal products offer us, many people are still afraid of animal fats. We need to overcome our heavily ingrained thinking that animal products are unhealthy and instead remember that animal fats provide essential nutrients for our bodies. Furthermore, keep in mind that man has been eating animal products since the beginning of time. We have genetically evolved to eat and benefit from the nutrients in animal products.

## What About Tallow?

Tallow—a saturated fat—was historically used for frying foods before processed vegetable oils came onto the scene. Tallow is rendered from beef the same way that lard is rendered from pork. What is rendering? It just means to melt something down. Tallow is 50% saturated fat, 42% monounsaturated fat, and only 4% polyunsaturated fat. Tallow is particularly high in a long-chain fat called stearic acid, which is the preferred fuel for the heart.

Unfortunately, tallow is rarely used now. For example, McDonald's corporation used to cook its French fries in a mixture of 93% beef tallow and 7% cottonseed oil before switching to 100% vegetable oil in 1990.[3] Remember, unlike the saturated fat found in tallow, the polyunsaturated fats found in vegetable oils do not hold up well to frying at high temperatures. Exposing vegetable oils to high temperatures causes them to oxidize. Oxidized polyunsaturated oils contain cell- and artery-damaging free radicals and can increase inflammation in the body that contributes to obesity, diabetes, heart disease, and cancer.

## What About Lard?

Lard is rendered fat from pork. This is another fat that people have been making in their homes for centuries to use as a solid fat for baking and cooking. Lard and chicken fat both contain more monounsaturated than saturated fat. These animal fat sources can therefore be categorized as monounsaturated fats. When baking, lard is a great alternative to shortening—it hasn't been highly refined, denatured, or hydrogenated. So why not try making your next pie with lard?

We must emphasize again, though, that it's crucial to purchase and use animal products from healthy animals that are pasture-raised without hormones and antibiotics.

## Does Saturated Fat Clog Arteries?

The mainstream medical establishment would have us believe that saturated fat should be avoided because it causes atherosclerosis–in other words, it clogs arteries. But nothing could be further from the truth. Research has not supported this conclusion. In fact, scientists have found that atherosclerotic lesions contain much more polyunsaturated fat than saturated fat. Specifically, atherosclerotic plaques often contain 74% unsaturated fat and only 26% saturated fat, with 41% of that unsaturated fat being polyunsaturated fat![4]

## Does Saturated Fat Make You Fat?

Another fallacy of eating fat is that too much dietary fat will cause obesity. There is no credibility to that argument. Fat does not make you fat assuming that you are eating healthy, good fats. Here's what does make you fat: carbohydrates, sugars, processed foods and heavily refined and processed fats and oils.

Dietary fat provides satiety so that we feel full and are not hungry. Eliminating fat from the diet often leaves a constant state of hunger.

That constant, gnawing hunger often leads to binging on carbohydrates, which can lead to obesity. More about fat and weight in Chapter 8.

## What About Eggs?

Eggs are an amazing powerhouse of nutrients. They are a fantastic source of protein as they are the only whole food source that contains the full complement of all of the essential amino acids. Furthermore, eggs provide a good source of vitamins A and D, the B-complex vitamins, choline, biotin, folic acid, and potassium.

Over 40 years ago, The-Powers-That-Be declared that eggs were bad for us when they said that egg consumption caused elevated cholesterol levels and cardiovascular disease. Eggs fell out of favor and Americans began eating fewer eggs. Erroneously, many people turned to egg whites as an alternative...but the majority of nutrients in the egg are found in the yolk!

Remember that the nutrients in an egg are only as good as the environment in which the chicken was fed and raised. Chickens packed tightly in cages are under constant stress. This stress lowers their immune systems and raises their likelihood of infection. Many times, chickens are fed copious amounts of antibiotics to combat the high infection rate. Chickens are meant to be roaming outside and eating insects, not cooped up inside!

Compared to conventionally raised chickens, the eggs from pastured or free-range chickens are very different in taste and yolk color—they're more buttery-tasting, and their yolks are bright orange-yellow. Furthermore, free-range chickens provide eggs with a much higher nutrient value.

Note that color of shell plays no role in nutrient value—different breeds of hens lay different-colored eggs. Contrary to popular belief, brown eggs are not necessarily healthier than white eggs. For optimal nutrients, be sure to buy free-range, organic eggs from chickens not fed hormones or antibiotics. To find healthy eggs, find a local farmer near you at www.localharvest.com.

## What About Butter?

Butter is one of the best sources of healthy fats as well as the vitamins and minerals that support heart, brain, and bone health. It's a shame that many people avoid butter because they think margarine is a healthier choice (or because they think butter will make them fat). It is time to debunk that idea! Besides being an excellent source of fat-soluble vitamins, butter has many other nutritious properties, including being a good source of:

1. **Arachidonic acid–** needed for prostaglandin production
2. **Butyric and lauric acids–** have antifungal and antimicrobial substances
3. **Conjugated linoleic acid or CLA–** known for its anti-carcinogenic properties
4. **Lecithin–** needed to metabolize fat
5. **Trace minerals–** particularly selenium, which is an important antioxidant
6. **Short- and medium-chain fatty acids–** support the immune system and are used as energy

These are just some of the reasons that butter is a better food choice than margarine or shortening. Margarine is an industrially processed pseudo-food. It has excessive levels of trans fats and is one of the real contributors to heart disease.[5] Butter really is better!

Did you know that studies have shown that we can absorb the vitamins and minerals in vegetables better when we eat those vegetables with butter? That's because butter contains good fat, and we need fat to help absorb minerals. So go ahead and butter those green beans! You'll get more out of all of your veggies if you enjoy them with butter. Plus, butter helps our bodies convert plant carotenoids into vitamin A, so be especially sure to butter your red- and orange-hued vegetables like carrots, yams, and winter squashes.

One more tip: you could also sprinkle on some unrefined salt (like Redmond's Real Salt® or Celtic® Sea Salt) to make those buttered green beans taste even more delicious. And since sea salt contains a wealth of minerals, you'll benefit from the minerals in the green beans **and** in the salt. Talk about an added bonus!

## What About Tropical Fats?

Along with butter, The-Powers-That-Be love to portray tropical fats as bad fats because of their supposed "harmful" levels of saturated fat. Due to the proclamations that coconut and palm oil are unhealthy, we have considerably lowered our consumption of tropical oils over the years. Given that the mainstream medical establishment was wrong about butter, though, is it a surprise that they're also wrong about coconut and palm oil?

## What About Coconut Oil?

Coconut oil contains beneficial saturated fats—it can actually help with thyroid, hormonal, and weight issues. It's also rich in lauric acid, a certain type of fat with immune-enhancing properties. Many scientific studies have demonstrated that lauric acid has anti-bacterial, anti-fungal and anti-viral properties.

A form of lauric acid is found naturally in human breast milk. To a great extent, it's what helps prevent infants from being infected by viruses and bacteria. Coconut oil is one of the few fats containing this hard-to-find fatty acid. Palm oil is another one. Coconut oil is also high in capric and caprylic acid, both of which have been shown to be beneficial in treating Candida albicans or yeast infections.

Yet another unique aspect of coconut oil is that it's primarily composed of medium-chain fatty acids (MCFAs). MCFAs are quite stable when exposed to high temperatures and are therefore not prone to oxidation. As previously mentioned, that stability makes coconut oil a great oil to use when cooking—it can withstand high heat. Another bonus is that it doesn't require refrigerated storage.

Furthermore, our bodies digest and utilize MCFAs differently than other fats—we make use of them immediately as an energy source.

That's why they're great for weight loss. More about fats and weight loss in Chapter 8.

## What About Coconut Milk?

Coconut milk contains healthy fats. Unfortunately, it's another great fat that has gone by the wayside as people have reduced the fat in their diet. Coconut milk is the liquid that comes from the grated meat of the coconut. This is a very nutritious food and a healthy source of fat that can be used as an alternative to milk for those on a dairy-free diet (although it does not have vitamins A and D and other nutrients only found in milk and animal foods).

Coconut milk is thick and rich and can be used in smoothies and over oatmeal. This is a great way to get your dose of coconut oil daily—every 10.5 ounces of coconut milk yields about 3.5 ounces of coconut oil. Just don't confuse coconut milk with coconut water, which is a clear liquid from young green coconuts. Coconut water is also very beneficial due to its high potassium and mineral content, but it offers different nutrients than coconut milk. Coconut water makes a great energy/sports drink because it helps replenish electrolytes. It's a great alternative to unhealthy sugar-laden commercial sports drinks.

## What About Palm Oil?

Palm oil is a tropical oil that has also gone by the wayside (along with coconut oil) due to the brainwashing we have received about saturated fats from The- Powers-That-Be. While coconut oil has made a great comeback in recent years, palm oil has not gained the same momentum. Red palm oil comes from the fruit of the oil palm tree. Palm fruit oil contains mainly palmitic and oleic acids and is about 50% saturated. Palm oil has received a bad reputation due to the deforestation and unsustainable harvesting methods often used in its production. However, we suggest that you include sustainably harvested virgin organic palm oil in your healthy diet—it's packed with antioxidants such as carotenes and vitamin E and other phytonutrients important for good health.

## What About Olive Oil?

Olive oil—along with palm oil and lard—is rich in oleic acid or omega-9 fats. Unlike omega-3 fats and omega-6 fats, omega-9 fats are not considered essential since our bodies can manufacture omega-9 fatty acids. Other omega-9 fats and sources of oleic acid include almonds, macadamia nuts, peanuts, butter, sesame oil, peanut oil, avocados, cashews, sunflower oil, almonds, pistachios, hazelnuts, and pecans. Olive oil contains a large amount of oleic acid. Oleic acid is one of the main reasons why olive oil is so healthy since oleic acid is known to support the cardiovascular system and help reduce blood pressure.[6]

But not all olive oil is created equal! You may have heard of virgin or extra-virgin olive oil. Virginity refers to the purity of the final oil as well as how the oil is produced. Olive oil is one of the few oils that can be mass-produced without industrial processing, heating and deodorization methods that damage the oils (those damaging methods are used to produce vegetable oils like soy, safflower, and canola).

To make sure you're buying high-quality olive oil that has not been industrially processed or overheated, look for bottles of extra-virgin olive oil. The term "extra-virgin" means that the oil comes from the first pressing of the olives and that the pressing is done in cold, controlled conditions rather than high-heat refinement factories. Extra-virgin olive oil retains the olive's maximum flavor and aroma—one whiff, and you'll think you're in an olive orchard. High-quality olive oil has a peppery/buttery flavor that varies from bottle to bottle depending on the type of olive that was pressed to obtain the oil. If a bottle of olive oil does not say extra-virgin (or minimally virgin), you can be sure the oil was heavily refined and that inferior olives were used to produce the oil. Such an oil does not have any taste or smell and has lost most of its health-promoting nutrients.

Extra-virgin olive oil is chock-full of nutrients, phytochemicals, and antioxidants such as vitamin E that help prevent damage in our bodies caused by free radicals. Olive oil is said to have over two hundred micronutrients, all of which are important in the prevention of aging, osteoporosis, arthritis, stroke, heart disease, and cancer. And not only is extra-virgin olive oil delicious in dressings and spreads, it can be used in body-care products—it's good for our skin, too!

## What About Essential Fatty Acids?

As previously mentioned, EFAs are called "essential" because we cannot synthesize them in our bodies—we must get them from our food. Without these essential fatty acids, we can't survive.

EFAs (omega-3 fats and omega-6 fats) are an important part of a healthy diet. As we already know, a deficiency or imbalance of EFAs does not create optimal health. We need to make sure we are eating healthy types of omega-3 fats (from chia, flax, fish, cod liver oil, etc.) as well as healthy sources of omega-6 fats (from nuts and nut butters, unrefined oils like sesame oil, free-range/pastured animal products, or sometimes supplements like evening primrose oil or black currant seed oil). The following are just a few of the many benefits of EFAs:

1. Aid in the production of prostaglandins, which are hormones that regulate body functions such as heart rate, blood pressure, blood clotting, fertility, and conception. Prostaglandins also play a role in immune system function by regulating inflammation and encouraging the body to fight infection.
2. Ensure brain and mental function in both children and adults.
3. Manufacture and repair cell membranes in our brains, eyes, ears, testes, ovaries, adrenals and the membranes that surround and protect every cell in our bodies.
4. Produce hormone-like eicosanoids that regulate immune and inflammatory responses.
5. Provide proper growth in children, particularly when it comes to neural development and maturation of sensory systems. It's especially important that fetuses and breast-fed infants have access to EFAs through their mother's dietary intake of EFAs.
6. Support for cardiovascular, reproductive, immune, and nervous systems.

## Do I Need More EFAs in My Diet?

That's a tough one since the answer will vary from person to person. Unfortunately, as discussed in Chapter 3, the Standard American Diet (SAD) contains too **many** of a certain kind of EFAs, namely the adulterated and poor-quality omega-6 fats that are found in highly processed sunflower, safflower, canola, corn, and soy oils (which is what you're getting when you buy a bottle of refined vegetable oil). Keep in mind, there are also too many omega-6 fats in common supermarket items such as eggs, fish, meat, and dairy products from factory-farmed animals.

On the flip side, omegas-3 fats are sadly lacking in the Standard American Diet, and when they are present, they're often damaged. That's because much of our food has been subjected to heavy processing and refining. For example, think about the cereal aisle in a typical grocery store. Those boxes of extruded, high-heat-processed flakes are designed to last forever. The so-called "heart-healthy" omega-3 fats they boast about on the label were damaged during processing, and since omega-3 fats oxidize very quickly, they don't have a long shelf life. Hence, they're often missing or damaged in a diet focused on processed foods.

As our society has turned more and more to highly processed "convenience" foods, our dietary imbalance of omega-6 to omega-3 fats has become more and more prevalent. It is important to eat a good balance of EFAs, including both omega-6 and omega-3 fats.

## What Is a Balanced Omega-6:Omega-3 Fats Ratio?

As we mentioned previously, the typical American is eating an unhealthy ratio of omega-6 to omega-3 fats that falls somewhere between 10:1 and 20:1.[7] (Plus, remember that many of the omega-6 fatty acids being consumed by Americans are of very poor quality since they have been hydrogenated, highly refined, bleached, or deodorized.) A much healthier ratio would be a ratio somewhere between 2:1 and 4:1 omega-6 to omega-3 fatty acids. To achieve the proper ratios, it is important to avoid conventionally raised animal foods, highly processed foods and refined oils. Table 6 shows you the omega-6:omega-3 ratios for common oils. Notice that most of these oils (except for flaxseed and walnut) are significantly higher in omega-6's and need to be avoided. Instead, purchase good-quality fats and oils as well as meats, eggs, and dairy from organic free-range/pastured animals whose products have the proper ratios of omega-6 fats and omega-3 fats that our bodies need.

**TABLE 6: Omega-6:Omega-3 Ratios For Common Oils**

| Oil | Ratio |
|---|---|
| Canola | 22:1 |
| Corn | 83:1 |
| Cottonseed | 256:1 |
| Flaxseed | 1:4.2 |
| Grapeseed | 690:1 |
| Peanut | No omega 3 |
| Safflower | 186:1 |
| Sesame | 138:1 |
| Soybean | 8:1 |
| Sunflower | No Omega 3 |
| Walnut | 4:1 |

## What is Wrong With Having Too Many Poor Quality Omega-6 Fats in the Diet?

Too many omega-6 fats can lead to inflammatory problems. Chronic inflammation is a problem because, over time, inflammation can damage healthy tissues. Common inflammatory diseases include asthma, rheumatoid arthritis, gingivitis, celiac disease, and Crohn's disease. Inflammation is also associated with obesity, diabetes, cancer, and heart disease as well as other conditions listed in Table 7.

**Table 7: Diseases Associated With Inflammation**

Asthma
Autoimmune diseases
Cancer
Cardiovascular disease
Celiac disease
Crohn's disease
Gingivitis
Heart disease
Irritable bowel syndrome & inflammatory bowel disease
Macular degeneration
Metabolic syndrome
Obesity
Psychiatric disorders
Rheumatoid arthritis
Type 2 diabetes

Decreasing our dietary intake of poor quality omega-6s so that we have a better-balanced ratio of omega-6s to omega-3s can greatly reduce the incidence of the many inflammatory conditions that plague Western societies. Omega-3 fatty acids—when eaten in proper balance with omega-6 fatty acids—have been shown to be efficacious in treating and preventing various diseases.[8]

## What About Fish?

Fish can be an excellent example of a good source of healthy fats, particularly omega-3 fatty acids. In particular, cold-water fish is high in the long-chain fatty acids EPA and DHA. These are what prevent fish and marine animals from freezing when they're swimming in cold waters. The fish we suggest consuming most often are species that are lowest in environmental contaminants, and that are eco-friendly and high in omega-3 fats. For example, wild salmon from Alaska (fresh, frozen, canned), albacore tuna (from U.S. and Canada), anchovies, Arctic char, Atlantic mackerel, sardines, and sablefish are all good choices.

We highly suggest you avoid farm-raised fish and instead only eat sustainable wild-caught fish. That's because wild fish contains a balanced ratio of essential fatty acids thanks to its natural diet of plankton and krill. The plankton and the krill are what contain the health-enhancing omega-3 fats, and when wild fish eat plankton and krill, these fish are rich in omega-3s fats, too. When we eat the fish that has eaten the plankton and the krill—well, you get the picture. That old saying is true: you are what you eat. According to The American Journal of Clinical Nutrition, farmed salmon has two to three times fewer omega-3 fats than their wild counterparts.[9] One of the best examples of wild-caught fish is Alaskan sockeye salmon.

Watch out for farmed salmon! Much like the sad state of animals on factory farms, farmed salmon is raised in pens where the fish are packed in very closely together. Too-tight living conditions mean higher chances of disease. In fact, most farm-raised fish are fed antibiotics to prevent infection. They're also often pumped full of hormones to make them grow faster and bigger.

If all of that weren't enough, here's the kicker: farmed salmon are fed color chips in order to make them look more enticing in the store. The pellets they're given to eat don't contain the pigments the fish would be eating in their natural environments, and those naturally occurring pigments are what gives salmon their lovely array of colors. Without the color chips, farmed salmon wouldn't be pink—it would be gray. The fish industry knows it cannot present farm-raised gray salmon for sale and expect to make profits.

In addition to avoiding farmed fish, it is important to steer clear of fish that may be highly contaminated with mercury, PCBs, dioxins and other chemicals. (Farmed salmon has been shown to contain up to 10 times more PCBs than wild salmon does.[10]) Aside from wild salmon, some other safer choices include sardines, herring, and anchovies. On the other hand, large fish that have high levels of contamination should be avoided. These fish include halibut, marlin, seabass, shark, swordfish, and walleye.

There is an ongoing controversy as to whether the benefits of fish outweigh the negative effects of heavy metals (e.g., mercury) and toxins (e.g., PCBs) consumed. We have found that taking supplements such as chlorella or alpha lipoic acid when eating fish helps to mitigate some of the negative effects of eating fish by binding the toxins. A great resource on fish can be found online at www.seafoodwatch.org.

## What About Nuts and Seeds as Well as Nut/Seed Butters and Nut/Seed Oils?

Nuts and seeds offer a host of EFAs as well as many vitamins and minerals. They tend to have more omega-6s than omega-3s and are also high in omega-9 fatty acids. (But recall that omega-9 fatty acids are not essential—they can be made in the body if necessary.) Table 8 lists just some of the healthy nutrients found in nuts and seeds. More information about nuts and seeds can be found in our book *The Guide to Healthy Eating*.

**Table 8: Healthy Nutrients in Nuts and Seeds**

**Almonds**—more calcium than any other nut, plus copper, iron, potassium, phosphorus, riboflavin, vitamin E, zinc
**Brazil Nuts**—calcium, manganese, phosphorus, selenium, thiamin, zinc
**Cashews**—iron, magnesium, phosphorus, potassium, zinc
**Hazelnuts**—calcium, copper, iron, magnesium, phosphorus, potassium, manganese, thiamin
**Pecans**—monounsaturated oleic acid, calcium, iron, magnesium, phosphorus, potassium, selenium, zinc
**Pumpkin Seeds**—iron, phosphorus, potassium, riboflavin, thiamin
**Sunflower Seeds**—folate, niacin, potassium, zinc

Many conventional doctors and dieticians feel that nuts may adversely affect cholesterol and lipid levels since they contain high levels of fat. However, their concern is not warranted, as nut consumption has been shown to lower elevated cholesterol levels and improve fatty acid profiles.[11 12] Our experience is that nuts can be used to help improve the lipid profile in patients.

Nuts as well as nut butters can also help build healthy immune and nervous systems. The nutrients found in nuts and nut butters provide the body with a wonderful source of protein and a quick source of energy. If you are buying nut or seed oils, be sure to buy cold-pressed or expeller-pressed oils and keep them in the refrigerator. These oils should not be used for cooking, but they're great for salad dressings and spreads. As far as nut butters, it is best to buy them raw and organic if possible. Please note, however, that due to nuts and nut butters being quite high in omega-6 content (as seen in Table 9) they should not be eaten excessively, but as a small part of a varied diet. Furthermore, when it comes to nuts and seeds in general, we suggest you buy them raw and soak and dehydrate them for optimal digestion and utilization of their nutrients. You can also then grind the nuts up for delicious homemade nut butters.

**Table 9: Omega-6:Omega-3 Ratios For Common Nuts/Seeds**

| Nut/Seed | O6:O3 Ratio |
|---|---|
| Almond | 28:1 |
| Almond Butter | 28:1 |
| Cashews | 44:1 |
| Peanut Butter | 176:1 |
| Pecans | 21:1 |
| Pine Nuts | 300:1 |
| Pistachios | 52:1 |
| Pumpkin Seeds | 119:1 |
| Sesame Seeds | 96:1 |
| Sunflower Seed Butter | 503:1 |
| Walnuts | 4:1 |

## What About Flax and Chia?

Flaxseeds and chia seeds are another option that stand out because they are both very high in anti-inflammatory omega-3 fats, specifically short-chain ALA. Short-chain fatty acids are what our bodies assemble into the long-chain fatty acids called EPA and DHA that we discussed in Chapter 3. Unfortunately, our ability to assemble these fatty acids can be compromised by stress, infections, alcohol, excess sugar and/or by vitamin or mineral deficiencies. These health-inhibiting risk factors are becoming more and more common as increasing numbers of Americans ingest too much sugar and refined food products. It is important to eat omega-3 fats in the form of both the short- and long-chain varieties.

Chia seeds are one of our favorite plant sources of short-chain omega-3 fatty acids. They are amazingly nutrient-dense and are one of the best plant sources of protein. Chia seeds are also a good source of calcium, manganese, and phosphorus. Chia seeds help boost energy, aid digestion and stabilize blood sugar. The seeds were once used by Aztec warriors as a running food in order to provide a quick energy source, and many athletes still use them today to provide better endurance.

Chia seeds are also rich in antioxidants that help protect the body from damage caused by free radicals, aging, and cancer. Chia seeds are easily digestible—they don't need to be ground up—and since they're mild in flavor, they can be added to pretty much anything. Both flaxseeds and chia seeds can be added into smoothies, sprinkled over oatmeal or stirred into yogurt. Because of the combination of protein, fiber, and their gelling action, chia seeds help you stay full longer and experience fewer cravings.

Flax, on the other hand, needs to be used with caution as it does have some phytoestrogen content and may disrupt hormone levels if used in excess. We suggest only using just a teaspoon or two of flax seed oil in salad dressings.

## What about Soy Oil?

Here we have also been led astray by The-Powers-That-Be. The short answer is that soy is not a healthy product and does not belong in the good fats category. Why? Soy has many anti-nutrients and can cause thyroid issues. The vast majority of today's soy products are made from genetically modified soybeans. Soy crops are sprayed with more pesticides than any other crop. And that's just the tip of the iceberg.

Frustratingly, soy has found its way into countless products on grocery store shelves. Be sure to read labels and avoid products containing soy oil, soy flour, soy protein isolate or any other derivative of soy. If you see an oil that is simply called vegetable oil, odds are that it contains soy. Soy oil as well as other vegetable oils are all highly refined, processed, deodorized, and chemically altered before they even reach the store shelf. Nearly all soy oils contain unhealthy, highly processed, deodorized, bleached, and refined fatty acids.

Since we do not recommend non-fermented soy in any form, in this book, we've categorized soy with the bad fats. We'll discuss soy further in the next chapter. Additional information on why soy is not a health food can also be found in our book *The Soy Deception*.

## The Final Skinny:

To achieve and maintain optimal health, good fats must be consumed on a daily basis. There is a lot of misinformation about fats continually repeated by The-Powers-That-Be. It is important to educate yourself about fat and understand the difference between good fats and bad fats.

As a general rule, processed vegetable oils and hydrogenated oils—as well as the fats and oils found in processed food sources such as bread, pasta, and cereal—are not good-quality fats. Good-quality fats are found in whole food sources and in animal sources (meat, eggs, butter, tallow, lard) when the animals have been allowed to eat a healthy diet. Other good fats include tropical oils like coconut and palm oil as well as olive oil, nuts, and avocados. See the *5 Steps to Optimal Health with Good Fats* in the back of this book to guide you in including good fats in your diet as well as the recipes in Chapter 12.

So-called "heart-healthy" oils such as soy oil and margarine do not supply healthy fats for our bodies and should be avoided. The next chapter will delve into these and other bad and ugly fats we suggest you avoid at all costs!

## (Endnotes)

1 Masterjohn, Chris. Adjuncts to the Fat-Soluble Vitamins, Published online 28 January 2013, "http://www.westonaprice.org/fat-soluble-activators/nutritional-adjuncts-to-the-fat-soluble-vitamins".

2 *Fed Proc* July 1978 37:2215.

3 Schlosser, Eric (2001). *Fast Food Nation: The Dark Side of All-American Meal*, Houghton Mifflin, ISBN 0-395-97789-4.

4 *Lancet*, 1994 344:1195.

5 Gillman M.W., et al. Margarine intake and subsequent coronary heart disease in men, Epidemiology, 1997 8(2):144–149.

6 Proc Natl Acad Sci U S A., 2008 September 16; 105(37): 13811–13816, Published online 4 September 2008. doi: 10.1073/pnas.0807500105.

7 Kris-Etherton P.M., Taylor D.S., Yu-Poth S., Huth P., Moriarty K., Fishell, V., Hargrove R.L., Zhao G., Etherton T.D.. Polyunsaturated fatty acids in the food chain in the United States. Am J Clin Nutr 2000;71:179S-188S.

8 Am J Health Syst Pharm., 2009 Jul 1;66(13):1169–79, doi: 10.2146/ajhp080411.

9 "http://usatoday30.usatoday.com/news/opinion/editorials/2002-10-06-oplede_x.htm. Accessed 2.7.14".

10 "http://usatoday30.usatoday.com/news/opinion/editorials/2002-10-06-oplede_x.htm. Accessed 2.7.14".

11 Am.F. Clin. Nutr., 2002 Nov;76(5):1000.

12 J.Nutr., 2001. Sep;131 (9):2275.

# 5

# Fat: The Bad and Ugly

**Now that you have learned about saturated fats and essential fats**, there's something else you should know: there's more to a healthy diet than just eating those health-enhancing good fats. Think of what's needed to maintain a healthy budget. There's more to budgeting than just depositing money in an account, right? After all, if you don't pay attention to how much you spend, you can spend more than you deposit and wind up with nothing in the bank.

Food is like finance for the diet. You need to consider the whole picture in order to maintain good health. When it comes to food, along with embracing the good fats, we need to avoid the bad and the ugly fats. In other words, keep depositing those good fats, but don't run out and buy bad ones!

We covered the good fats, so now let's talk about the bad and the ugly fats. Unfortunately, it's not difficult to find bad fats since many healthy foods that naturally contain good fats are remade into low-fat or no-fat products of questionable nutritional value or processed products that often contain unhealthy bad and ugly fats (such as polyunsaturated fats that were once healthful but have been damaged and made rancid by industrial processing methods.) These altered foods are not what we've historically eaten as human beings. These are the bad fats. Do we really think we can side-step evolution and Mother Nature with our "heart-healthy" fat substitutes and expect to be healthy?

Not all fats are created equal. Good fats, in fact, are not "created" at all—they already exist in nature. Food scientists and chemists have spent decades trying to duplicate nature and create low-fat alternatives and fat substitutes that, unfortunately, don't have anywhere near the nutritional value of the fats they're supposed to replace. Furthermore, these alternative foods often have increased levels of salt, sugar, and/or refined grains to make up for lost flavor and texture.

In the 1960s and 1970s, the polyunsaturated vegetable oil industry jumped on the low-fat bandwagon to fund, sponsor, and promote the use of vegetable oils as they helped discredit saturated fats and animal fats. Not only do these man-made substitutes lack nutrients, they have gone through harmful extraction methods, high-heat refining, and chemical processing, all of which lead to devitalized products. Devitalized food products are bound to cause deterioration in our health as well as lead to disease, weight gain, and cancer. In fact, devitalized polyunsaturated oils have been shown in studies to promote tumor growth.[1]

Let's look at the most common oil found in nearly every supermarket across North America: vegetable oil. This generic label is often applied to corn, soy, safflower, and sunflower oils. These oils are heavily refined, purified, and chemically altered. During the refinement process, these oils are rendered rancid, and that rancidity can cause free-radical damage to blood vessels and body cells. This kind of damage often leads to arteriosclerosis and cancer (among other diseases). Some research shows cancer can't occur unless there are unsaturated oils in the diet.[2]

Remember margarine? Once promoted as the miracle of fat substitutes, we were told, "Don't eat butter, eat margarine to save your heart." Now, even the food industry has been forced to recognize that margarine is full of harmful trans fats and is not heart-healthy. Those ugly trans fats actually inhibit the ability of our cells to utilize healthy fats. This causes a host of undesirable side effects, such as immune system dysfunction, heart disease, obesity, and cancer.

Trans fats will be discussed later in this chapter. We suggest you use this part of the book as a guide to help you go through your pantry and refrigerator and find any "heart-healthy," "low-cholesterol," "low-fat," "non-fat," hydrogenated, or processed oils that might be lurking in your kitchen. It's time to renovate!

## What Are "Bad" Fats?

Bad fats are fats and oils that have been subjected to very high heat, a laundry list of chemicals and extended processing. The end product is rancid and oxidized before it even hits the shelf at the grocery store, yet food manufacturers label these products as healthy. Most refined oils are made from polyunsaturated oils, which are delicate to begin with—they are the least suited oils to withstand high heat without becoming damaged. Processed and refined vegetable oils have become staples in many Western homes and most restaurants.

The oil refinement process ensures that the end product will create free radicals in the body. You're probably thinking that the term "free radical" sounds unduly dramatic. It isn't. It's actually a very fitting term considering the damage they cause. Basically, free radicals are molecules that are missing an electron. That makes them very unstable. That missing electron also makes free radicals extremely reactive, because they're constantly trying to "steal" electrons from other molecules to balance themselves. When they do manage to grab an electron, then the victim molecule is destabilized and turned into another free-radical thief. It's an endless loop of stealing and destabilizing. Free-radical damage to blood vessels and body cells leads to premature aging, arteriosclerosis, autoimmune disorders, and cancer, just to name a few conditions associated with it.

Given the havoc free radicals wreak on our bodies, we suggest you limit, or—even better—avoid bad fats entirely. Examples of bad fats are shown in Table 10.

**Table 10: Sources of Bad Fats**

- Canola oil
- Grapeseed oil
- Low- and non-fat foods
- Low-fat and skim milk
- Refined, overheated, deodorized, rancid or oxidized vegetable oils (e.g., soybean, corn, safflower, sunflower, and cottonseed)
- Margarine
- Peanut oil (refined)
- Vegetable-oil-based salad dressings
- Vegetable-oil-based spreads

## What Are Refined Vegetable Oils?

Common commercially refined vegetable oils include: canola (also called rapeseed) oil, soybean oil, corn oil, sunflower oil, safflower oil, and cottonseed oil. Refined vegetable oil starts with the seeds of various plant sources. Highly intensive mechanical and chemical processes are used to extract the oil from the seeds. During this processing, high temperatures and pressures are used to extract the oil. Part of this process includes heat treatment with a solution of caustic soda and the use of nickel as a catalyst. Nickel is a heavy metal that is very toxic to the body and is known to cause cancer. Petroleum-based products such as hexane are used as solvent baths. Research shows that a hexane residue is left in the final product. In fact, in 2001, the U.S. Environmental Protection Agency issued regulations on the control of emissions of hexane gas due to its potential carcinogenic properties and environmental concerns.

Finally, if that wasn't enough, the oil goes through deodorization to remove the horrible odor and taste that result from the industrial processing methods. Removing the odor means that consumers will no longer be able to detect the rancidity of the oils by their taste or smell. (When an unrefined oil becomes rancid, it's obvious—you can taste and smell the rancidity, at which point you know it's time to get fresh oil.) Some of the other various processes these oils go through are bleaching, degumming, emulsification, fractionation hydrogenation, interesterification, and neutralization. We find it preposterous that these highly processed oils are labeled as healthy oils.

## What Is Wrong With Refined Vegetable Oils?

Since refined vegetable oils are polyunsaturated oils, they are very unstable when subjected to heat, light and/or oxygen. Omega-6 fats and especially omega-3 fats are very sensitive to modern food processing. The high temperatures and pressures that occur during the refining process remove all of the naturally occurring nutrients such as vitamins and antioxidants. However, there is more bad news. The oils also become more toxic and dangerous to our bodies because processed oils contain more of the dangerous free radicals that do damage to our cells.

If that weren't enough, in order to prolong shelf life, the food industry often removes the omega-3 fats during the processing phase since they would quickly oxidize and this results in a product with a shorter shelf life. This means, of course, that processed oils lack the benefits of the omega-3 fats that should have been present in the oil and **are** present in the unrefined versions of these oils.

According to Mary Enig and Sally Fallon of the Weston A. Price Foundation, "High-temperature processing causes the weak carbon bonds of unsaturated fatty acids, especially triple unsaturated linolenic acid, to break apart, thereby creating dangerous free radicals. In addition, antioxidants, such as fat-soluble vitamin E, which protect the body from the ravages of free radicals, are neutralized or destroyed by high temperatures and pressures. BHT and BHA, both suspected of causing cancer and brain damage, are often added to these oils to replace vitamin E and other natural preservatives destroyed by heat."[3]

It's possible to destroy the benefits of these delicate oils at home, too—you don't want to use high heat with polyunsaturated fats as they cannot withstand high temperatures without forming free radicals. These oils should never be heated, and they should be stored in the refrigerator to keep them as fresh as possible.

## What About Canola Oil?

Canola is often touted as being a healthy oil, and it's found in many prepared foods as well as in many "heart-healthy" recipes. In order to prevent heart disease, we're told that canola is the healthiest cooking oil that we can use and that it's equally nutritious as an alternative to olive oil in salad dressings. The-Powers-That-Be and many scientists have endorsed canola oil, saying it's a "heart-healthy'" oil that's low in saturated fat, high in monounsaturated fat and is a good source of omega-3 fatty acids. But you've already learned enough from reading this book to know better.

First of all, there is no such thing as a canola plant. Canola was developed from the rapeseed plant. Rapeseed is inherently high in a toxic compound called erucic acid. The erucic acid levels in rapeseed are so high that it isn't edible, although rapeseed oil is fine for industrial/factory uses. In order to transform rapeseed into an edible oil, Canadian scientists genetically modified the rapeseed to remove the erucic acid and increase the levels of oleic acid. ("Canola" stands for "**Can**adian **o**il, **lo**w **a**cid.")

Nowadays, with its high oleic content, canola is advertised as a "healthy" oil for cooking and baking. And it's in many processed foods, too. But in many cases, the already-genetically-modified canola oil is also hydrogenated and consequently is high in trans fats. (We will discuss more about hydrogenation and trans fats later). Rather than benefitting us, the omega-3 fatty acids that we think we're getting from canola have been made rancid by the hydrogenation process. That means those once-helpful fats are actually harmful. Furthermore, canola oil—like all polyunsaturated oils—cannot withstand high temperatures. Heating canola oil allows free radicals to form. Refined canola oil is therefore rancid before it even hits the store shelves.

## What About Soybean Oil?

Most people are confused about soy. The soy industry and the media would have you believe that soy is a healthy alternative to dairy. They would have us believe that soy is a miracle food and that ingesting soy can help overcome illness as well as enable optimal health. Furthermore, they want us to believe that soy formula is a good choice for infants. Unfortunately, all of these ideas are false. Soy contains many anti-nutrients and components that are toxic to humans. Processed soy like soybean oil is **not** a health food.

Soybean oil has become the world's most widely used "edible" oil in part because it can boast that it is lower in saturated fat than animal fats. According to the United Soybean Board 2009 Consumer Attitudes Report, consumers ranked soybean oil among the top three healthy oils; in the United States, soybean oil is the most frequently consumed oil.

Oil sold as vegetable oil is often 100% soybean oil, and most restaurants use soybean oil for cooking and frying. Since soy is also a commodity crop and is therefore inexpensive to produce and purchase, soybean oil is found in many consumer products including margarines, spreads, dressings, sauces, and other items (see Table 11).

**Table 11: Items That May Contain Soybean Oil**

| | |
|---|---|
| Bakery items | Processed foods |
| Canned foods | Salad dressing |
| Coffee creamer | Sauces |
| Cooking oil | Shortening |
| Margarine | Spreads |
| Mayonnaise | Vegetable oil |

Soy is not a "health food" as the soy industry would have you believe. The truth about soy is that it has many toxins, anti-nutrients, and enzyme inhibitors. But what about the Japanese? They eat lots of soy, and they're healthy, right? The truth is that soy is not eaten in Asia the way it's eaten in America. In traditional and modern Asian cultures, soy products are fermented before being eaten. Fermented soy is produced by a host of bacteria, molds, and yeasts making it healthier for human consumption. Common fermented forms of soy include miso, natto, tempeh, and fermented soy sauce (e.g., shoyu or tamari). The fermentation of soy significantly reduces the anti-nutrient and anti-thyroid compounds and increases the health-promoting probiotics, the "good" bacteria, such as lactobacilli to enhance our intestinal health. Americans, however, generally eat non-fermented soy in the form of soybean oil, soy flour, soy milk, soy burgers, etc. Non-fermented soy is not healthy and has been linked to many health issues such as breast cancer, digestive problems, hypothyroidism, infertility, and thyroid cancer.

The soy industry has a vested interest in promoting wider uses of soy. However, there is a dark underside to the soy story that shines a different light on soy. The soy industry does not want the negative effects of soy exposed. For more about why we suggest you don't consume soybean oil or any other types of unfermented soy, see our book *The Soy Deception*.

## What About Unrefined Polyunsaturated Vegetable Oils?

Not all polyunsaturated oils are bad. As mentioned in Chapter 4, several polyunsaturated oils are health-enhancing, especially when the oils are unrefined/cold-pressed/expeller-pressed and when they're used as part of a varied, whole-foods diet. Unrefined oils such as sesame, pumpkin seed, or flaxseed oil are examples of healthy polyunsaturated oils that can be used in a healthy diet. Also, supplements like black currant seed oil or evening primrose oil are beneficial for our health.

Tragically, however, most polyunsaturated oils found in grocery stores have been subjected to damaging high temperatures, refining, processing, and chemical extraction, which means that these oils are already rancid and oxidized before they even hit the shelves. These are not good items for your pantry!

Examples of food containing rancid polyunsaturated fats include: most processed foods, salad dressings, spreads and all items containing refined corn, safflower, sunflower, and cottonseed oil as well as soybean and canola oil. You'll notice that these oils are colorless, tasteless, and odorless. That's because these heavily processed oils are often deodorized and bleached to remove their rancid smells and sludgy appearances. They're also high in omega-6 fatty acids. Remember the importance of consuming a good balance of omega-6s and omega-3 fatty acids? Overeating polyunsaturated oils that are mostly comprised of omega-6 fatty acids can lead to imbalances in the omega-6:omega-3 ratio and can lead to inflammation and/or disease. Plus, most of the omega-6 fatty acids in these food sources are of poor quality to begin with because they have been subjected to hydrogenation processes and/or have been highly refined.

## What About Low-Fat and Non-Fat Foods?

Since two-thirds of Americans are overweight or obese, many people are trying to lose weight by choosing low-fat and no-fat foods. And even people not trying to lose weight erroneously think that low-fat and no-fat foods are a healthier choice. But despite claims made by The-Powers-That-Be and the 20-billion-dollar-a-year diet industry, low-fat and no-fat foods are not healthy for you. One reason is that when you take out the fat, you take out the flavor as well, which means that low-fat and no-fat foods typically contain added sugars and/or chemicals to make the product taste better. Then there's the fact that low-fat, high-carbohydrate diets can lead to diabetes, insulin resistance and metabolic syndrome. More about this issue in Chapter 7.

In our experience, we've found that patients who eat low-fat foods often resort to eating a diet comprised mostly of high-carbohydrate foods. This leads to constant hunger pangs. Hence, a low-fat diet can predispose people to eat more carbohydrates and sugar—all because they're avoiding fat. The end result is weight gain and a difficult time losing weight.

Adequate dietary fat is necessary for good health. We have seen very few patients who thrive on a low-fat diet; most patients who primarily eat a low-fat diet have many metabolic markers in disarray. As we discussed in Chapter 4, dietary fat provides satiety as well as helping with the absorption of many nutrients.

## What About Low-Fat or Skim Milk Products?

Low-fat and skim milk products are not healthy foods, either. For one thing, when the fat is missing, the beneficial fat-soluble vitamins A and D are missing, too. To compensate for this, the dairy industry adds synthetic versions of both vitamins A and D. (Artificially added vitamins A and D are not as nutritious as the A and D that were originally in the full-fat milk.) Also, dairy producers almost always put powdered milk in low fat/skim milk to give these products the texture and mouth-feel that would normally come from the natural fat.

The issue with powdered milk is that it is highly oxidized due to the high-heat methods used to turn the milk from a liquid to a powder. Powdered milk contains oxidized cholesterol. Cholesterol itself is not bad for you, but oxidized cholesterol is. Oxidized cholesterol is the type of cholesterol that is linked to heart disease.

If you choose to eat dairy, we suggest you use organic dairy sources and buy the full-fat versions. Cultured forms of dairy are much healthier for you—kefir and yogurt are great choices. Optimally, you want to source your dairy from a local farmer and opt for raw or low-heat-pasteurized versions of your dairy products in order to obtain optimal nutrients and digestibility. That said, keep in mind that many people cannot tolerate dairy in any form. For more about this issue we refer you to our book, *The Guide to a Dairy-Free Diet*.

Now you know about the good fats from Chapter 4. The good fats are unrefined, unprocessed fats; these include monounsaturated, polyunsaturated, and saturated fats. The bad fats consist of any fat that has been refined and processed (such as rancid polyunsaturated vegetable oils). But we also have a third category of fat to explore: the ugly fats.

## What Are the "Ugly" Fats?

The "ugly" fats are the hydrogenated oils, trans fats, and also the inter-esterified fats that have no place in our food supply or in our bodies. These ugly fats cause hormonal imbalances and weight gain and can lead to many illnesses, including heart disease and cancer. Table 12 lists the ugly fats and the foods that contain ugly fats. For your own health, please completely avoid these!

**Table 12: Ugly Fats**

- Hydrogenated oil or partially hydrogenated oil
- "Heart-healthy" spreads
- Interesterified fats
- Margarine
- Shortening (e.g., Crisco)
- Trans fat

## What Is Hydrogenation?

Hydrogenation is a process that transforms liquid vegetable oils into solid fats. This industrial process forces hydrogen atoms into unsaturated oils (usually polyunsaturated vegetable oils) with the help of a metal catalyst, often nickel or platinum or copper. The nickel catalyst can also contain 50% nickel and 50% aluminum. These metals remain in the end products and therefore are present in food made from these products. It's worth noting that aluminum has been associated with Alzheimer's and other neurological diseases.[4]

This process also involves adding emulsifiers and starches for better end consistency. Finally, steam-cleaning methods and bleaching alters the unappetizing sludgy color, changing it to a more appetizing neutral white. Then the hydrogenated oil is put into tubs and sold as a foodstuff or is used as an ingredient in other foods. However, the end product is anything but healthy.

## Why Is Hydrogenation Used?

The process of hydrogenation was invented to alter the chemical structure of oils to increase their shelf life and to make cheap spreadable products similar to butter. Hydrogenation is an inexpensive process that uses low-cost commodity oils to create huge profits for manufacturers. During World War I and especially during World War II, butter was in extremely short supply, yet people still wanted it for cooking and baking. Hydrogenation had become possible in the 1800s, but it didn't take off until wartime demands made butter so scarce. Crisco and margarine are common examples of hydrogenated oil. Most hydrogenated oils today are made from soy oil. Items labeled as being partially hydrogenated mean that all of the double bonds are not completely saturated with hydrogen. These items are still not healthy choices for you. We consider hydrogenated and partially hydrogenated fat sources to be "ugly" fats.

## Why Are Hydrogenated Oils Bad for Our Bodies?

Hydrogenated fats/oils interfere with the body's ability to absorb and utilize good fats. During hydrogenation, liquid vegetable oils become solid and artificial new fatty acids are formed. These toxic fatty acids, known as **trans** fatty acids, are foreign to our bodies, and they lead to a host of problems. Among other things, they interfere with the body's utilization of natural fatty acids.

Although hydrogenated products were originally promoted as being healthier than conventional butter, ever since the 1990s, researchers and doctors have been realizing that hydrogenated fats have deleterious health effects. Hydrogenated fats have been associated with a host of health problems, including cancer, diabetes, heart disease, degenerative conditions, autoimmune disorders, thyroid conditions, and digestive problems. Most of these diseases were exactly the diseases we were trying to avoid when we started eating these "heart-healthy" fats. As we said previously, you're better off with butter!

## What Are Trans Fats?

Trans fats are artificial, man-made unsaturated fats which contain trans isomer fatty acids. Trans fats are much cheaper to produce than many natural saturated fats (butter, for example, or coconut oil). Trans fats are added to foods to enhance flavor, extend shelf life and improve texture. They are common in fried foods, commercial baked goods, processed foods and margarine. Trans fats are also found in foods such as microwave popcorn and frozen pizzas, refrigerated doughs, cookies, biscuits and ready-to-use frostings. They are also sometimes used by restaurants for frying. Many larger chains have phased them out, but smaller restaurants may still source ingredients containing trans fats from restaurant supply companies.

Although trans fats do naturally occur in small amounts in foods like meat, most trans fats are artificially created in a laboratory. Industrial trans fats have a different structure which can lead to adverse effects in the body. They may in fact increase the development of many different chronic diseases.[5]

## Why Are Trans Fats Bad for Our Bodies?

Trans fats harm our bodies because they trigger inflammatory responses in our bodies at a cellular level. Cells incorporate trans fats into the cell membranes. Once those trans fats are in place, they damage our cell function by interfering with proper chemical and hormonal reactions. In other words, messages can't get through, causing our systems to experience a communications blackout. Trans fats are so bad for our cells and our bodies that we classify trans fats as **ugly** fats.

## What if a Product Says It's Trans-Fat Free?

Just because the food label states "free of trans fats" does not ensure that the product is healthy. For example, Girl Scout cookies are now trans fat free, but that does not mean they are good for you. Labels can be deceiving when it comes to trans fats. In 2006, the U.S. Government established new labeling policies which required food producers to begin disclosing the amount of trans fat in their products. However, manufacturers are actually allowed to say "0 g trans fat " even when the end product contains 0.5g or less trans fat per serving. It's such a shame that "zero" does not mean zero. Since we tend to eat more than just one serving (especially when the serving size has been reduced to make the numbers work in a manufacturer's favor), we are eating plenty of trans fats.

As more research is being done on the harmful effects of trans fats, more and more companies and food chains are voluntarily reducing or eliminating the trans fat content of their foods so that they can claim they have healthy foods. The FDA is getting involved as well—the agency is considering banning trans fats completely in our food supply by passing legislation that would require companies to phase out trans fats entirely.

According to FDA Commissioner Margaret Hamburg, there is no safe level of consumption of trans fats. To date, only a preliminary determination has been made that a major source of trans fats—partially hydrogenated oils—will no longer be "generally recognized as safe" or GRAS. If trans fats are indeed removed from the FDA's list of GRAS ingredients, then partially hydrogenated oils will be subject to premarket approval by the FDA.[6] While this is a step in the right direction, the FDA still lumps trans fats together with saturated fat and cholesterol and suggests that Americans should reduce all three of these fats to have a healthy diet. Of course, we disagree with the FDA when it comes to saturated fats and cholesterol as they are not the enemies they are made out to be.

But remember, even if refined foods don't contain any trans fats, they **do** contain sugars, artificial sweeteners, additives, chemicals and/or dyes that all lead to poor health. "Free of trans fats" on a label does not mean a food is healthy. You can achieve the healthiest diet by buying whole, unprocessed foods and preparing meals in your home from ingredients you trust. Use the recipes in Chapter 12 as well as those in our other book, *The Guide to Healthy Eating*, to help guide your choices.

## How Do You Know if a Product Contains Trans Fats?

Check the ingredient label. If you see hydrogenated or partially hydrogenated oil in the list of ingredients—or margarine or shortening—the product contains trans fat. Many frozen foods contain trans fats, as do many commercial baked foods such as cookies, cakes, breads, and crackers. Often, prepared foods at the grocery store or food ordered in restaurants are cooked in hydrogenated oils. In short, processed foods contain the most trans fats, as do almost every fast food you can think of. While many of the larger chains have phased them out, the oils they are using instead such as soybean and canola are not healthy alternatives either. Until the FDA's ban on trans fats takes effect, trans fats can still be found in many foods. Table 13 lists foods that commonly contain trans fats.

**Table 13: Items That Commonly Contain Trans Fats**

| | |
|---|---|
| Baked goods | Frozen dinners |
| Baking mixes | Granola bars |
| Cakes | Ice cream |
| Candy | Margarine |
| Cereal | Microwave popcorn |
| Coffee creamer | Muffins |
| Cookies | Pancake mixes |
| Crackers | Pie crusts |
| Donuts | Pizza dough |
| Fast food | Potato chips |
| French fries | Salad dressings |
| Frosting | Soups |
| | Vegetable shortening and spreads |

## What About Margarine?

Margarine consumption is associated with several diseases, including heart disease and cancer. As we've mentioned, margarine is made through the damaging process of hydrogenation. Then there are the bleaches, dyes and artificial flavors that are used to make margarine look and taste the way it does.

Many consumers who are not particularly interested in their health but are looking for a good bargain choose margarine over butter since it's cheaper. But what they don't realize is that all they're getting for their hard-earned cash is harmful trans fats and a lack of the health benefits that butter offers, like vitamins A and D (not to mention the lack of rich flavor that butter offers!) Bargain-shoppers are inadvertently doing themselves harm. They'll end up harming their wallets in the long term too, since the money they could have spent on delicious butter will instead go to pay medical bills. We suggest you ditch the margarine and eat good ol'-fashioned real butter!

## What About "Heart-Healthy" Spreads?

The spreads advertised as "heart-healthy" are far from healthy for you or your heart. They are often full of processed, rancid vegetable oils, which means they are also full of free radicals that damage our tissues and cells. This is hardly a health food. Furthermore, the process often used to create many of these spreads—interesterification—is even worse than the aforementioned hydrogenation process.

## What is Interesterification?

Interesterification is another example of food scientists trying to make butter-like products out of vegetable oils. This process uses enzymes or chemicals to alter the molecular structure of a vegetable oil to turn it into fat with an indefinite shelf life. Interesterification is similar to the process that creates trans fats and also produces molecules that do not exist in nature. You can find interesterified fats in the same types of processed foods where you would find trans fats such as margarine, baked goods, or salad dressings. Any product that says "vegetable oil' may contain either interesterified fats or trans fats. If a product is labeled "0% trans fats" or "no trans fats" but is made from vegetable oils, it more than likely is made with interesterified fats. These products should be avoided completely! Again, why not just eat real butter?

## The Final Skinny:

Modern processing has created fats and oils that are detrimental to our health and waistlines. Avoiding these man-made "bad" and "ugly" fats is imperative to achieve optimal health. The more processing, heating or refining an oil has been subjected to, the less healthy it is to consume. Natural fats that are easily extracted from their sources are the healthy way to go.

Going back to the fat basics and choosing traditional food sources such as butter, tallow, olive oil, and coconut oil will help you gain your health back (and lose the weight). Use the *Know Your Fats Quick Reference Guide* at the back of this book to help guide you as you select between the good, the bad, and the ugly fats!

## (Endnotes)

1 Carroll K.K., Hopkins G.J., *Lipids,* 1979 Feb;14(2):155–8.
2 *C. Ip, et al.*, Cancer Res., 45, 1985.
3 Mary G. Enig, PhD and Sally Fallon, *The Skinny on Fats*, January 2000 19:02.
4 Int J Alzheimers Dis., 2011; 2011: 276393. Published online 2011 March 8. doi: 10.4061/2011/276393.
5 Adv Nutr, July 2011 Adv Nutr,vol. 2: 332–354, 2011.
6 http://www.cnn.com/2013/11/07/health/fda-trans-fats/.

# 6

# Cholesterol: Friend or Foe?

**For decades, cholesterol has been demonized** by The-Powers-That-Be. The American Heart Association, The American Diabetic Association, The American Academy of Dietetics and Nutrition as well as the government and Big Pharma have all repeated the same mantra: we all need to lower our cholesterol levels to the lowest possible numbers. The-Powers-That-Be have erroneously convinced the media and most physicians that cholesterol is an evil substance in the body that leads to atherosclerosis and heart attacks.

Over the last 60 years, have The-Powers-That-Be succeeded in their goal of lowering our cholesterol intake? The answer is a resounding "yes." Over this time period, our dietary intake of cholesterol as well as fats and oils has declined. Low-fat products have been substituted for healthy foods containing natural fats. Unfortunately, most of these low-fat food items contain high amounts of sugar, carbohydrates and refined (often hydrogenated) vegetable oils. Our consumption of these low-fat products has soared. However, following these new dietary guidelines has not resulted in a healthier society. In fact, the opposite has occurred: we are more obese, more diabetic and suffer from more chronic illnesses than we did before we switched to low-fat and low-cholesterol foods.

Ongoing research repeatedly demonstrates that cholesterol is **not** the cause of heart disease. In fact, cholesterol is an essential substance for each and every cell in the body. No cell can survive without adequate cholesterol levels, in part because cholesterol has both anti-inflammatory and anti-infective properties. In the case of heart disease, when there is damage to an artery wall, cholesterol is recruited to try to heal the damage to the artery. It's a protective substance—think of it as a bandage for the artery wall.

According to Meyer Texon, an M.D. in the Department of Forensic Medicine at the New York University Medical Center, atherosclerosis is not a lipid disease, as proven by the fact that atherosclerosis occurs when cholesterol levels are low, high, and in-between. In other words, there is no clear relation between cholesterol levels and arterial damage. Dr. Texon explains that indicting fat and cholesterol for hardening arteries is like accusing white blood cells of causing infection. In the case of heart disease and atherosclerosis, cholesterol is the "band-aid" that is brought in to heal lesions in the arteries.[1] To put it in layman's terms, consider firemen who respond to house fires. Just because firemen are **present** at every house fire does not mean that firemen **cause** those house fires.

Studies such as those done by Krumholz at the Department of Cardiovascular Medicine at Yale University found that elderly people with low cholesterol died twice as often from a heart attack as did elderly people with high cholesterol.[2] Fifty percent of all the heart attacks in the U.S. occur in patients with **low** cholesterol levels. For women, studies show that high cholesterol levels are associated with longer lives.[3]

Life is simply not possible without adequate cholesterol levels. Adequate cholesterol levels are necessary to optimize neurological function—without cholesterol, the myelin sheath around the nerves disintegrates, and nerve function is impaired. In addition to the crucial role it plays in neurological health, cholesterol has many additional and protective functions, including detoxifying our bodies and helping to protect us from infectious diseases. And remember, every one of the trillions of cells in the body requires an adequate supply of cholesterol to maintain the strength of the cell membranes. Cell membranes are all made up of a phospholipid bilayer that contains copious amounts of cholesterol. Cholesterol helps strengthen this two-part layer and decrease its permeability.

In this chapter, we will discuss what cholesterol is and how it functions in the body. We will also clear up misconceptions about cholesterol. For instance, contrary to what you have been led to believe, your dietary intake of cholesterol and fat does not have any significant impact on your serum (blood) cholesterol levels. Why? Because cholesterol is produced in the liver as well as in every single cell in the body, and if you don't consume enough cholesterol for your individual needs, your body will make more of it.

Because cholesterol is such a vital substance, our bodies have an intricate system of cholesterol production and transportation. These cholesterol carriers are called LDL and HDL cholesterol molecules. When cholesterol is sent out from the liver to the body, they're packaged in LDL molecules. When cholesterol needs to be brought back and recycled in the liver, it's returned by HDL molecules.

Now let's talk more about why low cholesterol is **not** optimal and why we need cholesterol to live.

## What Is Cholesterol?

The word "cholesterol" comes from the Greek word "chole" (meaning bile) and "steros" (meaning solid or stiff). Cholesterol is a fat-like substance produced in every cell in the body. Although it's often referred to as a fat, it is actually a waxy substance that belongs to a class of molecules called sterols. Most cholesterol is produced in the liver and, as previously stated, cholesterol is crucial to proper functioning of each of the trillions of cells in our bodies.

## How Is Cholesterol Transported Within the Body?

Since cholesterol cannot travel alone in the bloodstream, it combines with proteins to form small packages called lipoproteins. Lipoproteins are neat little bundles that contain fat (lipids) on their insides and protein on their outsides. There are two types of lipoproteins: high-density lipoproteins, or HDL, and low-density lipoproteins, or LDL.

Many people refer to LDL cholesterol as "bad" cholesterol and HDL cholesterol as "good" cholesterol. But LDL and HDL cholesterol molecules are neither good nor bad forms of cholesterol. They are produced in the body to transport cholesterol to the tissues and the liver, and each performs a valuable and necessary function. In a nutshell, LDL carries cholesterol from the liver to the cells, while HDL takes the cholesterol from the blood vessels and away from the cells and carries it back to the liver. Once in the liver, HDL is recycled, broken down or sent out of the body as waste.

## What Does Cholesterol Do in the Body?

Cholesterol is needed to build and maintain cell walls, repair damaged cells, make hormones, and create bile salts that help us digest fats. It also acts as an antioxidant to protect us from free radical damage. Cell membrane permeability and fluidity rely heavily on cholesterol.

Furthermore, the body uses cholesterol to make vitamin D. Vitamin D is necessary for maintaining healthy bones as well as for optimizing nervous system function. Also, insulin production, reproduction, and immune system health are all dependent on having adequate vitamin D.

Did you know that mother's milk is very high in cholesterol? Babies need it, too. Cholesterol is an important building block of the neuron pathways that are needed for healthy brain and nervous system development in children.

Cholesterol is a precursor to all adrenal and gonadal steroid hormones. These hormones include DHEA, testosterone, pregnenolone, cortisone, progesterone, and estrogen. Figure 8 shows the hormone cascade. As you can see, cholesterol is at the top since it is the precursor to all of them. These hormones are essential to life—without them, we would die. Looking at this chart, you can see that the adrenal and gonadal hormones depend on adequate cholesterol levels. Dr. Brownstein has written extensively on the benefits of maintaining optimal hormone levels. More information about this topic can be found in his book, *The Miracle of Natural Hormones*.

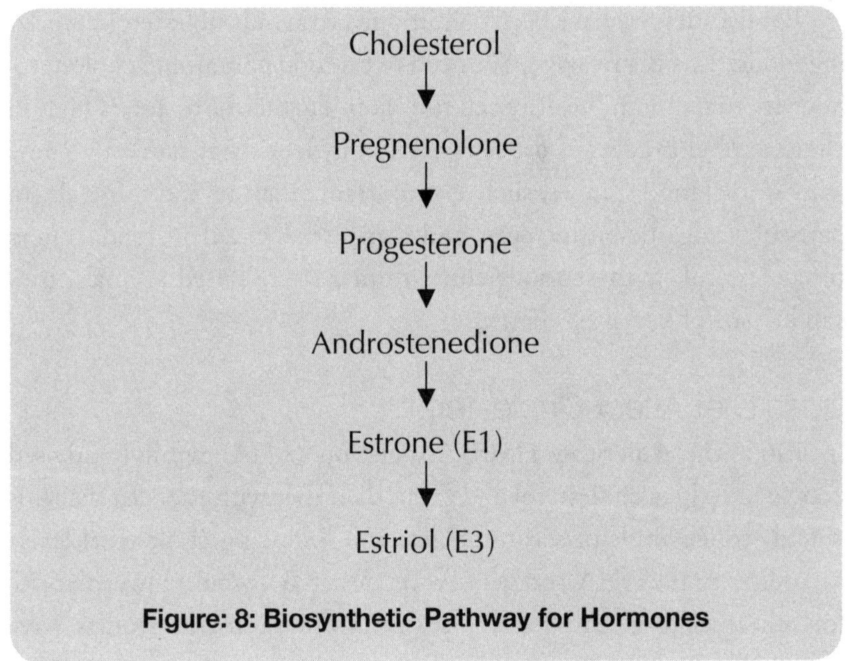


**Figure: 8: Biosynthetic Pathway for Hormones**

## How Does The Body Produce Cholesterol?

The liver is the organ responsible for producing the majority of the body's cholesterol. In addition, cholesterol is created by cells that line the small intestine and by individual cells in the body. Cholesterol is the essential substance needed to create all new cells, plus it's used to help repair injured areas of the body. Cholesterol also helps protect us against infection. Knowing these facts, you can see why studies have shown that low cholesterol has been found to be associated with an increased risk of dying from cancer, gastrointestinal problems, and respiratory infections.[4]

## What Foods Contain Cholesterol?

Cholesterol is only found in foods that are derived from animals. Any package of plain frozen peas that brags about containing "zero cholesterol!" is stating the obvious in the name of marketing. Butter, eggs, and red meat are examples of foods that contain cholesterol.

For decades, we have been conditioned to avoid cholesterol-containing foods. This is a mistake. We need to eat food containing cholesterol in order to maintain healthy cell function. Furthermore, foods high in cholesterol also contain other essential nutrients that naturally come with animal food sources, such as important vitamins and minerals. In particular, organic butter, eggs, and meat are all excellent food sources of cholesterol. If these foods come from pasture-raised animals, they can be part of a healthy diet.

## Does Diet Affect Cholesterol?

In 1965, the American Heart Association (AHA) wrongly advised people to reduce cholesterol and fat in their diet with the idea that this would reduce levels of serum cholesterol. Reducing cholesterol levels, according to the AHA and The-Powers-That-Be, would lower the risk for atherosclerosis and heart disease. However, major studies have shown that diet has little or no effect on serum (blood) cholesterol.[5 6] Remember, cholesterol is produced in the liver as well as by each and every one of the cells in the body. If you lower your dietary intake of cholesterol-containing foods, your body will adjust by producing more cholesterol. The inverse also holds true: if we eat more cholesterol, our bodies will produce less of it. In fact, according to Uffe Ravnskov in his groundbreaking book *The Cholesterol Myths*, our body actually produces three to four times more cholesterol than we eat.

## Does High Cholesterol Cause Heart Disease?

No. This is a sixty-year fallacy that has been promoted by The-Powers-That-Be. They say that lowering dietary cholesterol will lower the risk of heart disease, stroke and other cardiovascular disorders. As a society, we have followed their advice and drastically reduced our consumption of meat and eggs and other cholesterol-containing foods. However, research does not support that lowering the intake of animal products has reduced our risk of cardiovascular disease. Furthermore, lowering our cholesterol intake and eating more fat-free foods has not made us healthier! Instead, we have become obese and are facing an epidemic of chronic illnesses.

## Statin Drugs—Good or Bad?

This answer is easy! Statin drugs are bad. Statin drugs such as Lipitor, Zocor, Pravachol, and Crestor are the most profitable class of medications in history of Big Pharma. It's estimated that over 40% of American adults are currently taking a statin medication. They are one of the most commonly prescribed drugs in the U.S. Even children are now being put on these drugs.

Statins work by poisoning the enzyme HMG-CoA reductase. This enzyme catalyzes a reaction that allows cholesterol to be produced in the body. Statin drugs lower cholesterol levels by rendering this enzyme ineffective. So do statin drugs lower your risk for mortality? No—statin drugs have never been shown to lower mortality risks. Do statin drugs lower your risk for a heart attack? Not much. The best the statins have been shown to do is lower your risk of a non-fatal heart attack by about 1% **if** you have already had a stroke or a heart attack. However, the 1% reduction in risk is also only **if** you are a man between the ages of 39–59 years. For women, statins have never been shown to lower the risk for heart attacks. For those who have not had a cardiovascular incident—including both men and women—statins have never been shown to lower the risk of heart attacks.

How can statins be so widely prescribed despite not improving mortality rates? Statins are a classic example of good marketing and statistical manipulation by Big Pharma. Statins are associated with a host of serious side effects such as neurological disorders, brain fog and mental decline, cancer, liver problems, and muscle aches and pains. See Table 14 for additional adverse effects from using statins. Not only do statins not improve mortality, they just might shorten your lifespan. We think this is worth repeating: elevated cholesterol levels are **not** the cause of heart disease. More information about this topic can be found in Dr. Brownstein's book *Drugs That Don't Work and Natural Therapies that Do.*

**Table 14: Adverse Effects of Statin Drugs**

- ALS/ ALS-like syndrome
- Aneurysm
- Atrial fibrillation
- Autoimmune illness
- Breast cancer
- Cancer
- Cataracts
- CoQ10 depletion
- Diabetes
- Exercise limitations
- Guillain Barre
- Gynecomastia
- Heart failure
- Hepatic dysfunction
- Hepatitis B reactivation
- Hyperkalemia
- Hypertension
- Increased risk of infection
- Inflammatory myopathies
- Irritability/aggression
- Kidney damage
- Liver pathology
- Lupus
- Macular degeneration
- Memory loss
- Myalgia
- Myositis
- New difficulty walking
- Oroantral fistula
- Pancreatitis
- Parkinson's disease
- Peripheral neuropathy
- Prostate cancer
- Rhabdomyolysis
- Renal insufficiency
- Rippling muscle disease
- Sexual dysfunction
- Serotonin receptor depletion
- Skin cancer
- Sleep difficulties
- Tendinopathy
- Testosterone deficiency
- Thyroid disorders
- Weight gain

## What Are the Risk Factors for Heart Disease?

Many factors can elevate your risk of developing heart disease. Some of these include eating a poor diet, smoking, suffering from stress, having nutritional imbalances, and suffering from certain infections. Elevated cholesterol levels have been demonized as being the number-one cause of heart disease, but medical research does not support this idea. Half of all people who die from a heart attack have high cholesterol levels. That means the other half that die from a heart attack have low cholesterol levels.[7] In fact, high cholesterol may **protect** against infections and atherosclerosis.[8]

## What Are Good Cholesterol Levels?

Cholesterol levels measure how much cholesterol is circulating in your bloodstream. Elevated total cholesterol levels have been touted as being the culprit for heart attacks as well as indicators of whether you are at risk for having a heart attack. The-Powers-That-Be claim that a healthy cholesterol level is less than 200mg/dl. That is nonsense. Many people are perfectly healthy with a cholesterol level over 200mg/dl. In fact, during Dr. Brownstein's experience of 20 years of seeing patients, he has seen that the healthiest cholesterol levels range from 180–250mg/dl. Total cholesterol is **not** a very good indicator of your risk of heart disease. Not only that, but keep in mind that cholesterol levels naturally increase with age. Insisting that everyone's cholesterol level should not increase even as they age is ridiculous.

Unfortunately, mainstream medical professionals continue recommending lower target cholesterol levels. The only way to achieve these low levels is to use cholesterol-lowering medication. Even children are now being put on cholesterol-lowering medication. This is a disastrous policy—children need adequate amounts of cholesterol for proper neurological development. This trend is especially alarming when you consider that depression and suicide have been linked to low cholesterol levels.[9]

Who benefits most from lowered target levels of cholesterol? That answer is easy: the companies that sell statin medications. Following the cholesterol recommendations of The-Powers-That-Be would necessitate that the majority of Americans be prescribed a statin medication, despite the fact that these medications have never proven to prolong life or prevent heart attacks for the vast majority of people.

## Should I Avoid Fat and Cholesterol in My Diet if I Have High Cholesterol?

Again, we will say "No!" Before you agree with your doctor that your cholesterol is high, please read Dr. Brownstein's book *Drugs That Don't Work and Natural Therapies That Do* to gain a greater understanding of the subject. You will learn that our bodies naturally regulate cholesterol levels. That self-regulation makes it nearly impossible to raise cholesterol levels to very high levels by simply eating more cholesterol.

If your cholesterol level truly is too high, it is important to search for an underlying cause. Inflammation, toxicity, and infections can all raise cholesterol levels. In fact, in these conditions, an elevated cholesterol is the normal and expected response by the body. Taking a drug that blocks cholesterol production will not be beneficial. Rather than popping a statin pill, it's a good idea to identify and treat the underlying **cause** of elevated cholesterol levels.

Keep in mind the following facts about statin medications. Statins have never been shown to prolong life. Statins have never been shown to prevent a first heart attack. In women, statins have never been shown to prevent a heart attack or stroke. The best the statins have been shown to do is prevent a heart attack by approximately 1% in middle-aged men only if they have previously had a heart attack incident. In the elderly, statins have no proven benefits. The skinny on statins is simple: they are not the answer for anyone. Adverse side effects from statin drugs can be severe. These side effects include cognitive impairment, dementia, diabetes, neuropathy, and muscle damage.

## What About Obese People? Is Their Cholesterol Too High?

This is somewhat complicated. Yes, obese people can see their overall cholesterol, LDL cholesterol, and triglyceride levels increase. However, the elevated cholesterol numbers are not the cause of the obesity; they are the consequence of it. In other words, the elevated cholesterol numbers are the body's way of trying to cope with excess fat on the body. Excess abdominal fat is highly inflammatory. When people are obese, their bodies produce an anti-inflammatory molecule to try and cope with the excess adipose tissue. This molecule is cholesterol. Your body is trying to protect you, not kill you!

When it comes to obesity, understanding the underlying causes is paramount in order to develop a plan to reverse the process. This is the proper and prudent course of treatment.

## Can Cholesterol Get Too Low?

Yes, it is possible to have insufficient levels of cholesterol in your body. Cholesterol levels under 160mg/dl are associated with a host of serious medical conditions, including cancer and heart disease. The Honolulu Heart Study showed that patients with the lowest cholesterol had the highest mortality rates.[10] These results have been repeated dozens of times.

What we also haven't been told is that having low cholesterol levels decreases our protection against infection. In addition, remember that every single cell needs cholesterol to thrive. This includes brain cells. Cholesterol specifically affects the metabolism of serotonin, a substance involved in the regulation of your mood. It is no wonder that many neurological disorders such as Parkinson's and Alzheimer's are associated with low cholesterol levels. Here are just some of the additional issues associated with low cholesterol (less than 160mg/dl):

- Increased anxiety and suicide[11]
- Increased cancer, chronic fatigue, infections, and stroke[12] [13]
- Increased depression and bipolar disorder[14]
- Increased rates of school suspension[15]
- Increased violent behavior and aggression[16]
- More likely to become addicted and have more difficulty in kicking drug addiction[17] [18]

Many doctors and The-Powers-That-Be are telling their patients they need their cholesterol levels to be below 200 mg/dl. However, these doctors are missing the boat if they continue prescribing medications that lower cholesterol levels without searching for the underlying problems that cause cholesterol to rise in the first place. Cholesterol is a vital substance in the body; we cannot live without it. Cholesterol is not the villain it's made out to be–rather, cholesterol is needed to heal injured tissue, maintain cell integrity, as well as for many other critical functions in the body.

## What About Triglycerides?

Triglycerides (TGs) are the form that fat takes in our bodies and in the food we eat. TGs are a combination of a glycerol molecule and three molecules of fatty acids. Often doctors will measure your TG levels along with your cholesterol levels. This is called a "lipid panel test."

Similar to high cholesterol many people wrongly believe high TGs result from eating too much fat, this is not the case. Triglycerides are actually made by the liver when we eat too much sugar, fructose, as well as starchy and refined carbohydrate foods. Our bodies also wind up with too many TGs when we're under stress, when we smoke and when we suffer from infections. One way to reduce TGs is to clean up your diet and, in particular, reduce your sugar and carbohydrate intake (including alcohol). Also, detoxifying the liver is very helpful for hypertriglyceridemia. Dr. Brownstein and his partners have developed a detoxification product called Total Liver Care (TLC). More information about TLC can be found in Appendix B.

## The Final Skinny:

Don't be fooled by The-Powers-That-Be when they recommend eating low-fat foods to have low cholesterol levels in your blood. Fat and cholesterol are not the enemies. Cholesterol is made in the body because it is a health enhancing substance critical for many important functions in the body. For instance, it is a precursor to steroid hormones and Vitamin D, as well as being imperative to cell membrane integrity and cell communication. It is best to eat a healthy diet...which includes healthy sources of fat and cholesterol!

Remember, statin medications are the most prescribed medications in the history of Big Pharma! Chemically lowering cholesterol levels with a statin medication has never been shown to prolong life, but statins have been shown to have many adverse side effects. With the knowledge you gain from this book, you can make the best healthcare decisions for you and your family.

# (Endnotes)

1 "http://www.ncbi.nlm.nih.gov/pmc/articles/PMC1807837/pdf/bullnyacadmed00025-0020.pdf, Accessed 1.20.14."
2 Krumholz H.M. and others. JAMA. 272, 1335-40, 1994.
*3* *Lancet* Volume 333, Issue 8643, 22 April 1989, Pages 868–870.
4 Jacobs D. and others, Circulation 86, 1046–60, 1992, http://www.ncbi.nlm.nih.gov/pubmed/1355411.
5 Kannel, W.B. Kannel, W. B. and Gordon, T.: The Framingham Study. Diet and Regulation of Serum Cholesterol, Section 24, Dept. of Health, Education and Welfare, Washington, D. C., 1971.
6 Nicholas, A. B., Ravenscroft, C., Lamphiear, D. E., and Ostrander, D. E.: Daily nutritional intake and serum lipid levels: the Tecumseh Study, Am. J. Clin. Nutr. 29:1384-92, 1976.
7 Atherosclerosis, 149:181-90, 2000.
8 U. Ravnskov "http://qjmed.oxfordjournals.org/content /96/12/927.full. Accessed 2.4.14".
9 Epidemiology, 2001 Mar;12:168-72.
10 http://www.ncbi.nlm.nih.gov/pubmed/11502313.
11 J.Clin Psychiatry, 1994 Jun;55(6):252-4.
12 Chest, 2005;127:643-651.
13 Journal of Cardiology, 1998; 82:323-328.
14 Pediatr Res, 1994 May;35(5):602-10.
15 Am J Epidemiol, 2005;161:691-699.
16 Psychosom Med., 1994;56(6):479-84.
17 Drug Alcohol Depen, 1991 Dec 31;29(2):183-7.
18 Psychosomatic Medicine 65:86-91 (2003)

# 7

# Low Fat = High Carb

**One of the biggest issues with a low-fat diet** is that it ends up being a high-carbohydrate diet, which can lead to unwelcome blood sugar problems. Compared to people eating diets higher in fat, low-fat dieters are hungry more often and are prone to eating more carbohydrates, generally refined carbohydrates such as chips and snack bars. Unfortunately, many of these low-fat refined carbohydrate products contain added sugars to make up for the flavor and texture that are lost when the fat is taken out. In other words, when we avoid fat, we often wind up inadvertently eating more sugar. Not to mention the artificial colors, flavors, MSG and other flavor enhancers that are used to make low-fat products more palatable.

Because we have so much sugar in our modern low-fat-focused diets, many people develop both high and low blood sugar problems. That's because eating too much refined sugar can result in a rapid swinging of blood sugar from suddenly too high to suddenly too low. To combat these sudden bursts of heightened blood sugar, the pancreas releases copious amounts of insulin, an action which can result in a hypoglycemic (too low blood sugar) episode.

Hypoglycemia has become very common. Due to poor dietary habits, we are seeing more patients suffering from hypoglycemia as their blood sugar is on a daily rollercoaster ride of up-and-down, up-and-down. Hypoglycemia can negatively affect our brain, mood, and energy. Symptoms of hypoglycemia include amnesia, anxiety, apprehension, confusion, hallucination, irritability, and trembling. On the flip side, many people who are inadvertently eating too much sugar end up with type II diabetes because their blood sugar levels are consistently too high. Experts predict that the drastic increase of type II diabetes is one of the driving factors that is going to result in the current generation not outliving their parents for the first time in American history.

Let's get more specific about why a high-carb diet is a very bad idea. The most commonly consumed carbohydrates are in the form of sugars, refined grains and processed foods. Eating these on a regular basis leads to a host of problems, including weight gain and diabetes, two conditions which are closely linked. The average American eats 250 to 300 grams of carbs a day, accounting for about 55% of the average caloric intake. These numbers need to be significantly reduced—at least in half!—for weight loss to occur and to prevent type II diabetes. (Type II diabetes accounts for over 90% of diabetes cases in the U.S.) When we eat refined, simple carbohydrates like sugars and refined grains, our bodies release too much insulin, a condition called hyperinsulinemia. Hyperinsulinemia, in turn, often leads to insulin resistance and weight gain. Insulin resistance leads to diabetes. It's a nasty—but completely reversible—chain of events.

The best way to eliminate the hyperinsulinemia-to-insulin-resistance-to-diabetes sequence is to stop eating all those carbs and sugar and start eating a healthy, balanced diet that includes good fat and is full of nutrient-rich foods.

From a purely common sense point of view, we all instinctively know that fat is filling. As an example of this principle, try to eat more than one avocado. (The avocado, by the way, is full of good fat.) We bet you can't eat more than one whole avocado! But we're equally willing to bet that you could eat a large amount of chips and still be hungry. It's like the ad says: you can't eat just one. And therein lies the satiating power of fat. The fat-rich avocado will fill you up, while the carb-heavy chips will invite you to keep on eating. You might even eat the whole bag!

## How Does Insulin Work in the Body?

When we eat food, the digestive process breaks down the food into glucose. The glucose is used by the cells to make energy. Insulin is a hormone released by the pancreas in order to force the cells to take up glucose. All carbohydrates (this category includes sugars, of course) convert to glucose in the blood in order to supply the cells with the substance they need to produce energy.

All carbohydrates are not created equally. The more refined the carbs are, the quicker they convert to glucose. A piece of white bread will raise glucose and insulin levels higher than an apple will. Everything you eat comes with a different glycemic index number—that's a measure of how fast a carbohydrate turns into glucose in the body. Common examples of high-glycemic foods include white bread, white rice, white potatoes, beer, corn products and products containing refined sugars. Lower-glycemic foods are synonymous with good health. See the glycemic index chart in Appendix A.

If you continuously eat foods primarily made of refined carbohydrates, your pancreas will continue to pump out excessive levels of insulin to deal with the excessively high levels of glucose in your body. Soon, your cells become more and more resistant to insulin instruction even as your pancreas makes more and more insulin to push the same amount of glucose into the cells. This is called insulin resistance.

When people become insulin resistant, carbs become a bigger challenge for the body because the body has become tired of processing carbs and sugar. It begins to respond to them differently—instead of trying to push the glucose into the cells, the body stores the glucose in adipose tissues, or body fat. In fact, insulin is known as the fat-storage hormone.

People with metabolic syndrome most often have insulin issues and also have a large waist circumference that signifies this excess fat storage from excess insulin production. Furthermore, if people are insulin resistant for a long time, the pancreas gets exhausted and is unable to produce enough insulin to keep up with the glucose in the blood. That's when diabetes develops.

Interestingly, research has shown that consuming fats along with carbohydrate-rich foods helps reduce the glycemic impact on the body and therefore helps avoid developing insulin resistance and diabetes. Another great reason to include those good fats with every meal!

## What About Vegetarian or Vegan Diets?

We are not proponents of vegetarian or vegan diets. More often than not, vegetarians and especially vegans quickly become deficient in many nutrients. Also, these types of diets usually are focused mostly on carbohydrate-rich foods, which leads to many of the issues we have discussed in this chapter. Vegans in particular (vegans do not eat any animal foods) are often deficient in fat-soluble vitamins A and D, which can only be found in animal foods in a usable form. Many vegans believe they can get fat-soluble vitamins in plant foods. However, beta-carotene, the substance our bodies use to produce vitamin A, requires the presence of dietary fat in order for the body to absorb it, and not many plant foods are rich in fat.

This misguided thinking is what's going on with many biotech companies who are trying to improve nutrition in Third World countries. These companies are introducing products like the new genetically modified (GM) "Golden Rice," which contains more beta-carotene than traditional rice varieties and is meant to address vitamin A deficiencies. However, beta-carotene by itself is useless without fat![1]

## What About High-Fat Diets?

Fortunately, not all diet gurus have pushed an anti-fat agenda. Dr. Atkins, for example, seemed to have a good idea when he began promoting a high-fat, high-protein, low-carb diet. People following his non-fat-prejudiced advice lost weight and felt satisfied. The one big drawback of his plan was that he didn't put enough emphasis on seeking out healthy fats. As discussed in this book, healthy fats include unrefined plant-derived oils as well as animal products that come from animals raised on healthy, organic farms rather than in factory-farming operations.

People in many cultures have traditionally eaten high-fat diets, yet do not show the rates of heart disease or arteriosclerosis we would expect from that type of diet (if what we have been taught is in fact true). For example, the Maasai, who live in Kenya and drink about

5 gallons of whole raw milk every day and eat high-cholesterol food products do not have high cholesterol levels in their blood. Nor do the Maasai suffer from heart disease the way we do.[2] The Inuit, who live in the Arctic, traditionally got about 80% of their calories from fat. Similar to the Maasai, the Inuit who are pursuing their traditional diets do not suffer from heart disease and diabetes at the rates we do. Both of these cultures have been studied extensively and are proof that a diet high in unrefined, healthy fats does not lead to atherosclerosis or heart disease.

## The Final Skinny:

Low-fat, high-carb diets are not the way to go for optimal health and weight loss. They can create unwanted blood sugar issues in the body and also lead to diabetes. In fact, eating too little fat will stress the body and result in a lowered metabolism that will make your body prone to storing more fat. On the flip side, high-fat diets are linked to lowered blood sugar.[3] We suggest you eat more fat in order to lose weight and reach your optimal health! Learn more about eating fat to promote weight loss in the next chapter.

## (Endnotes)

1 "http://www.naturalnews.com/043774_Golden_Rice_GMOs_quack_science.html#ixzz2swKjNpHr. Accessed 2.10.14."

2 "http://sciencenordic.com/maasai-keep-healthy-despite-high-fat-diet, Accessed 2.8.14."

3 "http://www.eurekalert.org/pub_releases/2012-05/lu-hdl051112.php, Accessed 2.8.14."

# 8

# Eat Fat...and Get Skinny!

"Don't eat fat—it will make you fat."

"Don't eat fat—it has too many calories."

"Don't eat fat—it will clog your arteries and promote heart disease."

**Media "health experts" love to promote these erroneous claims** about fat. They—and we—have been hoodwinked by the mainstream medical establishment to believe that the less fat we eat, the better our health will be. But what if it wasn't true? What if fat does not make us fat? What if Julia Child was right when she said, "The only time to eat diet food is while you're waiting for the steak to cook!" and, "If you're afraid of butter, use cream." What if we should have been listening to Julia Child instead of the mainstream medical establishment all along?

Julia Child was right—it's a flat-out myth that all fats are bad. It turns out that unrefined, natural fats literally are the crème de le crème. Fat is an essential part of our diet. We cannot optimize our heath without eating fat. Our bodies need fat for many important functions, and if we don't eat enough healthy fats, we're likely to suffer from a myriad of health problems.

Unfortunately, most people—doctors included—are misinformed when it comes to dietary fat. The "all fat is bad for you" paradigm has been promoted for many years but has never resulted in its intended goal of improved health. Saturated fats, in particular, have been highly demonized. In the meantime, dieticians have assured us that polyunsaturated vegetable oils (corn, safflower, soy, sunflower, cottonseed, etc.) are heart-healthy, provide us with all of our fat-based nutritional requirements, and should replace saturated fats.

Over the last 60 years, we have significantly reduced the amounts of fat and saturated fat in our diet. But then why, during this same time period, have we become the most obese people to inhabit the planet? The reason is this: for the last 60 years, The-Powers-That-Be have been giving us the wrong advice when it comes to fat, and the consequences of following their recommendations to lower our fat intake have been disastrous. Two-thirds of Americans are overweight, and we now have more chronic, obesity-related health issues than we have ever experienced in our history as a nation.

Data from 2009 to 2010 shows that 17% of adolescents and children are obese. According to the National Institutes of Health (NIH), childhood obesity has become an epidemic. In addition, we're experiencing an alarming rise in the rate of type II diabetes.

We've been told by the medical and nutritional establishments to follow the advice issued by the U.S. Department of Agriculture (USDA) in the form of the food pyramid/MyPlate™. But even the new and "improved" MyPlate™ recommendations continue to do more harm than good for our health—the recommendations still teach people to follow a high-carb diet by focusing on low-fat foods. Plus, MyPlate™ combines saturated fats (the good guys) with trans fats (the bad guys) and tells us to avoid both.

From having read this book, you know the pitfalls of that advice! Now doctors recognize it, too. In a 2004 editorial in the Journal of American College of Cardiology, Sylvan Lee Weinberg, former president of the American College of Cardiology and an outspoken proponent of the diet-heart hypothesis, said, "The low-fat/high-carbohydrate diet, promulgated vigorously by the National Cholesterol Education Program, National Institutes of Health, and American Heart Association since the Lipid Research Clinics-Primary Prevention Program in 1984, and earlier by the U.S. Department of Agriculture food pyramid, may well have played an unintended role in the current epidemics of obesity, lipid abnormalities, type II diabetes, and metabolic syndromes."[1]

Why **aren't** these low-fat diet foods, fads, and weight-loss programs helping people lose weight or get healthy?

As we stated before, people on low-fat diets are constantly hungry and are prone to reach for quick foods containing high levels of refined carbohydrates. These refined sugars and grains cause people to have blood sugar issues. Fat is absorbed and digested much more slowly than carbohydrates, plus fat provides satiety. Carbohydrates do not. A high-carbohydrate diet results in wild fluctuations of blood sugar that lead to hunger cravings when blood sugar levels abruptly drop. The issues with low-fat, high-carb diets were previously discussed in Chapter 7.

Healthy unprocessed fat should be used to combat overeating. For obese people, although the numbers on the scale say that the body is overweight, the person is often undernourished, because most overweight people do not get enough nutrients in their diet. Fast food and processed foods do not offer the nutrients necessary for optimal health. When someone is overweight, it increases his/her health risks for many diseases, including obesity, diabetes, hypertension, cancer, and heart disease. (Collectively, these conditions are known as metabolic syndrome.)

A vicious cycle emerges as overweight people commit to low-fat diets. For one thing, as we have discussed in the previous chapter, low-fat inevitably means high-carb. High-carb is unsatisfying on many levels. Sugary foods lead to food cravings and overeating since the dieter never feels full, and often refined carbohydrates are consumed. These are rapidly turned into glucose in the body. Therefore, eating a carbohydrate-rich diet inevitably leads to blood sugar issues and often diabetes and/or hypoglycemia.

Many people look for low-fat foods, thinking that such foods are healthier choices. This idea could not be further from the truth. Low-fat foods are far from healthy; they should be avoided! Low-fat foods provide little nutrition...but they **are** full of unwanted additives, bad oils and fats (e.g. hydrogenated oils and trans fats) and artificial sweeteners and chemicals meant to enhance the taste of over processed foods. Ingredients found in low-fat foods can lead to hormone imbalances and weight issues. And do these low-fat foods ever taste good? No. It's the fat that makes foods taste good.

Many people cannot stay on low-fat diets for very long because they cannot withstand the constant feeling of hunger. According to a 2006 study reported in The New England Journal of Medicine, most people who participate in weight-loss programs "…regain about one-third of the weight lost during the next year and are typically back to baseline in three to five years."

Although Americans spend $40 billion a year on weight-loss programs and products, part of the answer is right in front of them. If someone is looking to lose weight, what he/she should do is make lifestyle changes rather than going on diets or joining weight-loss programs. It's important to eat a healthy and balanced diet, which means avoiding refined carbohydrates and sugars. Look for whole foods rich in nutrients, and also include plenty of natural, healthy fats. These fats will provide a feeling of satiety. That satiation will fend off food cravings and will decrease the tendency to overeat and overindulge. Put simply: in order to stop being tired, hungry, and overweight, it's time to start eating fat.

## Can Eating Fat Actually Help With Losing Weight?

First of all, remember that eating the wrong fats—that is, damaged and rancid fats like trans fats and vegetable oils—is harmful and can hinder weight loss. But also remember that not eating enough good fats hinders weight loss efforts as well. This is because when the body is starving for fat, it puts the body into a stressful state. In that case, the body will actually try to hold onto fat to make sure it has enough energy stores to survive.

One healthy fat in particular for weight loss and boosting metabolism is coconut oil. This tropical oil has been ostracized for containing saturated fat, but now we know that saturated fat is not the problem. Coconut oil is extremely beneficial and one of the healthiest fats you can include in your diet. Coconut oil is great for cooking and baking and is known for its immune-enhancing properties. Moreover, coconut oil helps protect against heart disease, cancer, and degenerative conditions. And yes, coconut oil even helps us lose weight thanks to its metabolism-boosting and thyroid-supporting properties.

Coconut oil is different than most fats in that it is made up of mostly medium-chain fatty acids (MCFAs). MCFAs are very stable—they don't break down and oxidize when heated. That makes coconut oil great for cooking and baking. Also, coconut oil does not need to be refrigerated. MCFAs are also digested and utilized differently than other fats in the body—they are used immediately to make energy in the body, which makes them great for weight loss.

According to Bruce Fife, ND and author of *The Coconut Oil Miracle*, "One food that can rev up your metabolism even more than protein is coconut oil. MCFAs [medium-chain fatty acids] shift the body's metabolism into a higher gear, so to speak, so that you burn more calories. This happens every time you eat MCFAs. Because MCFAs increase the metabolic rate, they are dietary fats that can actually promote weight loss."

It is important to buy good-quality virgin coconut oil. You will know you have a good oil if it has a nice flavor and is pleasant enough to eat by the spoonful. Virgin coconut oil is minimally processed so as to retain all of the coconut aroma and flavor. If you do not like coconut flavor look for expeller pressed coconut oil. Be sure to avoid coconut oil that has been refined and deodorized—this kind of oil will have little to no taste or smell. Refined coconut oil does not have the health benefits discussed in this book. For more tips and information about coconut oil, see the *Coconut Oil Quick Reference Guide* in the back of this book.

## The Final Skinny:

The right kind of fat can help you lose weight. Trans fats and low-fat foods should be avoided. Coconut oil can be a wonderful addition to your healthy food regimen. Coconut oil has medium-chain fats that have immune-enhancing factors, anti-infective properties and metabolism-stimulating effects that may even help you lose weight. Regularly consuming coconut oil can enhance anyone's diet!

## (Endnotes)

1 *J Am Coll Cardiol.*, 2004;43(5):731–733. doi:10.1016/j.jacc.2003.10.034 http://content.onlinejacc.org/article.aspx?articleid+1133027.

# 9

# Your Brain on Fat

**The famous Greek physician Hippocrates said**, "Whatever is good for the heart is probably good for the mind." He was right—not only is fat a healthy food for the heart, it is an optimal food for the brain!

Did you know that the human brain is over 60% fat by weight? So it's not surprising that fat is an essential nutrient for optimal brain health. In fact, more and more research is beginning to show the benefits dietary fats have on brain health and our day-to-day mental state.

Your daily diet affects the brain chemicals that in turn influence your mood and behavior. And there's even more: cognitive function, mental acuity, behavior, focus, and clarity all depend on consuming adequate amounts of dietary fat. Eating a low-fat diet can lead to depression, an inability to focus, behavioral illnesses (e.g., ADHD and ADD) and more.

However, remember that there are good and bad fats for your brain as well as your body. As we have discussed in this book, The-Powers-That-Be claim that all dietary fats are bad for us to ingest. They make no distinction between saturated fats and trans fats; for example, they state that both are bad fats. In this case, The-Powers-That-Be are wrong. Our brains, in fact, **do** need adequate amounts of saturated fats and EFAs to function optimally.

At the same time, eating bad fats can have a negative influence on brain function. That's because every cell membrane, the brain included, requires fat to function optimally. Simply put, if you eat bad fats, you will wind up with bad fats lining your cells. This leads to malfunctioning cell membranes throughout your entire body. And poor cell membranes will negatively affect all biological functions in the body, the brain included.

Choosing the right fats can make a big difference in not only how your brain functions but also how you feel. This chapter will explain why it's so important to eat good fats (including saturated fats) to ensure a healthy brain and a positive mental state.

The majority of the fat in the brain is saturated fat. Without this saturated fat, our brain cells would literally starve. Oleic acid, a monounsaturated fat, is also highly concentrated in the brain. It is a fatty acid found in olive oil.

The brain also contains polyunsaturated fats, namely those in the form of omega-3 fats. Omega-3 fats promote mental clarity, concentration, and the ability to focus. Studies have shown that omega-3 fatty acids are essential for maintaining normal cognitive function.[1] The long-chain fatty acids from the omega-3 family include EPA and DHA, and these are very prominent in the brain. They're crucial for properly functioning cell membranes and optimal brain function.

DHA is particularly abundant in our brains, even more so than EPA. Without DHA, cognitive function can become impaired. DHA bolsters our overall health and protects our brain cells. DHA and EPA are both so important for brain function that they are required ingredients in infant formulas in order to ensure proper brain, nerve, and eye health of growing infants.[2] EPA has also been found to help regulate mood, and it is an essential ingredient for combatting depression and mental disorders.

An imbalance in EFAs in the brain has been linked to hyperactivity, depression, and other mental disorders. What balance are we talking about? The delicate interplay of omega-6 fats to omega-3 fats we talked about in Chapter 3. Both fats have an important role to play, but the brain needs a 1:1 to 4:1 ratio of omega-6 fats to omega-3 fats. The typical American diet has a ratio of at least a 20:1 due to our culture's reliance on highly processed foods.

Keep in mind that the majority of omega-6 fatty acids in the Standard American Diet (SAD) come from highly processed vegetable oils and hydrogenated fats. These are unhealthy sources of omega-6 fatty acids. Processed food containing refined ingredients generally lack omega-3 essential fats. Furthermore, meat and dairy from factory-raised animals which are fed an imbalanced diet are far too high in poor-quality omega-6 fats. The key is to have the right balance of fatty acids for optimal brain function as well as for other functions in the body.

By now you've probably realized that when you avoid fat, you are starving both your brain and body. Remember, much of the outer membranes of our brain cells are made up of fats and cholesterol. Let's take a closer look at how our bodies convert the fats we eat into essential building blocks for our brains, bodies, and overall health.

When you digest the fats in your food, your body breaks the fats down into fatty acid molecules of various lengths. Your brain then uses these raw materials to assemble the special types of fats that it needs into its cells. The cells are a crucial part of the body's messaging system since all nerve signals must pass through the fat-rich cell membranes. Think of cell membranes as the mini-brains of each of our body's trillions of cells—the membranes evaluate the conditions of the environment surrounding each cell and then communicate what needs to be done to keep each cell powering along at optimal efficiency. A cell membrane that has poor-quality essential fatty acids cannot perform optimally and will cause overall brain function to suffer.

Another important task of the cell membranes is to serve as cellular gatekeepers by regulating the flow of nutrients and limiting the exposure of toxins. As learning and memory forge new connections between nerve cells, new membranes must be formed to complete those connections. The job of the membranes never ends.

All brain cell membranes continuously need to refresh themselves with a new supply of fats. That's understandable given that they have such a big job to do and that our brains oversee a much larger nervous system. Aside from giving us the ability to think, our nervous system transmits information and signals via neurons to cells throughout our body. Neurons are like small wires that transmit data to and from the brain. (Think of them as telephone wires. Without that wiring, there is no communication.) The protective coating surrounding the neurons is known as a myelin sheath. This sheath insulates the neurons and plays an important role in the communication processes. And guess what? The myelin sheath is composed of 15–30% protein and 70–85% fat. Some of that fat in the myelin sheath is cholesterol.

That brings us to another crucial-yet-controversial substance: cholesterol. It's one of the most important substances in our brains. We already know that cholesterol is needed for many functions, including making more brain cells. In fact, half of the white matter in our brains (which contains the nerve axons that allow for transmission of brain signals) may be composed of cholesterol-rich myelin.

Research has shown that there is a direct correlation between the concentration of cholesterol in the myelin and how well the brain functions. The myelin sheath facilitates nerve conduction by enabling information to get from the brain to our various body parts (or vice versa) almost immediately. When the myelin sheath is damaged, the transmission of information slows down drastically, which can lead to adverse consequences.

Multiple sclerosis is an example of an illness that can occur as a result of defective myelin sheathing. People affected with MS cannot carry out simple movements like writing or walking. According to the National MS Society, a diet higher in essential fatty acids may also help reduce symptoms of MS.[3] This again proves the point that healthy brains rely on good fats.

We know, too, that infants need cholesterol for proper brain development—that's why breast milk is so high in cholesterol. On a very basic level, cholesterol is needed to hold cell membranes together and to help them keep their proper shape. Cholesterol also maintains the vital components needed for cell receptors, which, in turn, are an essential part of the body's overall communication system. This is true for everybody, adults and children alike.

One of the worst things you can do for brain function is to take a statin drug that lowers your cholesterol level. It is no wonder that statin drugs are associated with a host of neurological side effects, such as brain fog, amnesia, and fatigue.

Remember too, fat makes up 70–85% of the myelin sheath. A very low-fat diet will not supply the myelin sheath with the raw materials it needs to repair and regenerate itself. Researchers have discovered that neurons without myelin—also called "gray matter"—process information at slower speeds. Other examples of disorders caused by damage to the myelin sheath are shown in Table 15.

**Table 15: Examples of Disorders Characterized by Damage to the Myelin Sheath**

- Acute disseminated encephalomyelitis
- Charcot-Marie-Tooth disease
- Devic disease (neuromyelitis optica)
- Guillain-Barre syndrome
- Leukodystrophy
- Multiple sclerosis
- Optic neuritis
- Pernicious anemia
- Transverse myelitis

Did you know that essential fatty acids and cholesterol are essential components of the entire nervous system? Both are necessary for our bodies to make and metabolize neurotransmitters such as serotonin, GABA, and tryptophan. Neurotransmitters are substances involved in mood regulation. As mentioned in Chapter 6, it's no wonder that many neurological disorders associated with aging (such as Parkinson's and Alzheimer's disease) as well as other behavioral disorders like violent tendencies, depression, and suicide are associated with low levels of cholesterol in the body.

To achieve optimal brain health, it is important to focus on foods that are rich in good fats and cholesterol. It's equally important to avoid processed foods such as commercial meats and dairy—those contain poor-quality omega-6 fats and lack omega-3 fats, and such foods do not promote a good balance of those fats in our bodies. In addition, we need to eliminate refined sugars and trans fats from our daily diet. It's also worth pointing out that when your diet is high in trans fatty acids and low in omega-3 fatty acids, your brain absorbs twice as many trans fatty acids. That is not a good situation for the brain.

So what should you and your family eat for a healthy brain? Focus on a balanced diet and meals full of healthy protein, carbs, and fats from organic sources whenever possible. Find a local farmer whom you can trust to provide you with the healthiest food possible. Visit www.localharvest.org to find local farmers (and farmer's markets) near you.

Also remember that your diet should include foods that are high in healthy fats. That means omega-3 fats and omega-6 fats along with saturated fats. Examples of food containing essential fats as well as many other important nutrients include chia seeds, flax seeds, wild-caught cold-water fish, eggs, and other animal products from grass-fed/free-range animals.

High-quality cod liver oil provides DHA and EPA so that your body doesn't need to go through the process of converting short-chain omega-3 fatty acids into long-chain DHA and EPA. This oil should be taken under a doctor's supervision to ensure proper fatty acid balance.

Finally, keep in mind that trans fats should be avoided at all costs! These highly refined fats are found in fast food, processed foods, margarine, French fries, commercial baked goods, many fried snack products (such as potato chips) and more. These trans fats are **not** good building blocks for a healthy brain—instead, they impair brain function. Trans fats have been so highly refined that they have become non-foods—that is, a material so foreign to our digestive systems that our bodies just don't know what to do with it. As a consequence, not only do trans fats interfere with normal fatty acid storage and metabolism, they disrupt proper communication in our brains. Trans fats become incorporated into our brain cell membranes, including the myelin sheath that insulates neurons.[5] This leads to a disruption of our communications systems as well as a decline in cognitive function.

Another unwelcome side effect of trans fats is that they have an unfortunate tendency to displace the good fats—that is, the saturated, oleic acid, and DHA fats that are the principal fatty acids in the myelin. If the good fats are not able to be where they should be and cannot do what they should do, cell-to-cell communication and activity can suffer. This compromised situation contributes to neurodegenerative disorders such as multiple sclerosis (MS), Parkinson's, and Alzheimer's.

Also, trans fats work against our brains by disrupting the production of energy in the mitochondria of our brain cells. Mitochondria are the energy factories of our cells. Plainly put, if you don't have the right amount of fats available, energy-producing cells cannot produce optimal amounts of energy.

## The Final Skinny:

Optimal brain function depends on fat and cholesterol. In fact, our brains are over 60% fat. It's important to eat good fats in the diet, including saturated fats from free-range/grass-fed animals. It's also crucial to consume foods offering the proper balance of omega-6 fats to omega-3 fats in order to optimize brain function. Low-fat diets can make you feel unwell and unhappy on a daily basis as well as limit the long-term potential of your brain and body!

# (Endnotes)

1 http://archive.ahrq.gov/clinic/epcsums/o3cognsum.htm.
2 http://www.redorbit.com/news/health/1314336/recommendation_infant_formula_should_include_omegas/.
3 "http://www.nationalmssociety.org/living-well-with-MS/health-wellness/nutrition, Accessed 2.12.14."

# 10

# Fats and Children

**One of the key issues under debate** is what a deficiency of fats and essential fatty acids does to our health, especially to our children's health as they grow and develop. Why is dietary fat so important for children? The answer is that adequate amounts of fat are essential for the growing brain. As we learned in Chapter 9, the brain is 60% fat by weight. The childhood brain will not develop normally when deprived of fat. Our national obsession with low-fat diets has caused many pregnant women and women of childbearing age to become deficient in fats and fat-soluble vitamins. A pregnant woman's deficiency will lead to a deficiency in her children.

Many children begin life with nutritional deficiencies. These deficiencies only worsen as they are fed the Standard American Diet (SAD) of low-fat and high-sugar foods. Since the neurological system is mostly made of fat, eating a low-fat diet is not helpful for a developing child. It is no wonder so many kids now have behavioral and emotional issues!

The food many children eat today is highly processed, low in fat and lacking the high-quality nutrients that are found in unprocessed eggs, meat, fish, fruit, nuts, seeds, and vegetables that come from natural sources. Unfortunately, the SAD **does** provide our children with a wide variety of poor-quality fats that have been hydrogenated and contain trans fats and/or fats that have been processed and therefore contain free radicals. Unrefined good fats and oils are often missing from children's diets today. Let's take a look at a few common meals.

For many children, a typical breakfast consists of skim milk and processed cereal that's usually made with refined wheat and contains as much as 40% added sugar by weight. This meal is often accompanied by a tall glass of orange juice or other fruit juice that is mostly just sugar. Whole fruit contains fiber, antioxidants, and is a fresh source of vitamins and minerals, but juice only contains the sugar component of the original fruit.

A SAD lunch might consist of macaroni and cheese made with refined pasta and over processed and rancid fats, additives, and dyes. Or lunch could be a sandwich on refined white bread, served with a box of juice containing plenty of sugar along with artificial colors and flavors. Dessert might be a cookie made with refined flour and copious amounts of refined sugar.

If that weren't already enough, the SAD often includes an afternoon snack of commercial goldfish crackers. These often contain MSG, refined flour, additives, and colorings. And again, these are often served with sugary fruit juice.

Finally, it's time for dinner. The SAD often consists of fast food or pizza made with refined flours, too much sugar and a large helping of highly processed meats and/or cheeses, all washed down with soda pop (i.e., sugar and chemicals). And then it's time for dessert again!

This SAD is a recipe for disaster for our children. Eating the SAD ensures our children will develop essential fatty acid deficiencies and will lack basic nutrients such as vitamins, minerals and enzymes.

The growing child's brain does not need or benefit from processed sugars, food chemicals, or additives such as glutamates that are neurotoxins–substances that can be poisonous to the brain and can negatively affect behavior. Neurosurgeon and researcher Russell Blaylock, M.D. has written extensively on this subject. His research has clearly shown that neurotoxins such as MSG and glutamate negatively affect the behavior and brain function of children. In his research, he points out that soon after MSG was adopted by the entire food industry there became obvious symptoms of "MSG syndrome," in which people affected would have flushing of the face, heart palpitations, and episodes of GI discomfort and diarrhea to name a few. Furthermore, his research showed that silent damage was also occurring to the brain in which there were few symptoms. Over time, he saw destruction of major portions of the brain, which could cause Alzheimer's, Parkinson's, and other brain ailments."[1]

Moreover, not eating enough good fats when neural pathways are being formed can lead to behavior issues and dysfunction such as ADHD. The fetus' neurological system forms during the first trimester. If the pregnant woman does not have an adequate supply of essential fatty acids to pass on to the developing fetus' brain, the brain will not develop normally. Similarly, a growing child needs a consistent supply of essential fatty acids to aid the brain in its growth and development phase. We have no doubt that we are seeing an epidemic of ADHD due to the SAD.

In addition to the lack of good fats in the SAD, as we've touched on in previous chapters, the SAD is far too high in refined carbohydrates, especially sugars. These instantly digested sugars turn into glucose in the blood. According to research by Stephanie Seneff, Senior Research Scientist at the Computer Science and Artificial Intelligence Laboratory at MIT, excess dietary glucose has severe ramifications for children as well as adults. When there is plenty of glucose but very little fat in the foods we consume–which is what happens when people eat low-fat, high-sugar foods–the muscles consume the glucose first, leaving the brain in the lurch, so to speak. The brain is deprived of the fats it needs to construct high-quality long-distance neural connections. In other words, a fat-starved brain cannot build a good communications system. Without a good communications system in place, everything breaks down.[2]

In children diagnosed with ADHD, many have been found to have shrunken white matter in the part of the brain that is involved with focus, attention, and the ability to acquire new knowledge. The brain changes may be due to an insufficient supply of good fats during the growth and developmental phase of the brain, when neural pathways are being formed.[3]

If we want to reverse the ADHD epidemic that has taken root in this country, we must change our thinking about dietary fat. The rates of ADD (attention deficit disorder), ADHD (attention deficit hyperactivity disorder) and other behavioral issues in our children continue to rise unnecessarily. Unbelievably, the Centers for Disease

Control and Prevention (CDC) estimates that 11% of all U.S. children are suffering from ADHD. Adults have similar difficulties in focusing on essential day-to-day activities, too—approximately 5% of U.S. adults suffer from ADHD.[4] [5] As a result, the CDC estimates that the total cost for ADHD is well over $50 billion annually.[6]

What exactly is ADHD? Put simply, it is a neurobehavioral disorder in which a person is not able to focus his or her attention on a task. People with ADHD are overactive, impulsive and unable to control their behavior. Ritalin is the number-one prescribed treatment for ADHD. But is this medication actually solving the problem? Do these patients have a Ritalin-deficiency syndrome? Of course not. Patients suffering with ADHD have imbalances in their nutrients, especially essential fatty acids. They often are eating low-fat, high-sugar diets, diets which further compound the core problem.

What we need to remember is that the brain needs key nutrients for proper development. Without those nutrients, we can infer that proper development may be delayed, interrupted, or—in the worst cases—never realized.

Now that you have a better idea of the valuable role fats play when it comes to our children's health, growth, and development, you can come up with an simple action plan to make sure you make better choices for your children. Get rid of fat-free products, including fat-free milk and yogurt. Enjoy whole milk and whole-milk yogurt, preferably organic and/or raw if available. Find resources for raw milk at www.realmilk.com.

Get rid of margarine and other butter substitutes and put butter back into the fridge. Butter contains a wide range of essential fats; substitutes do not. Skip the egg whites in favor of whole eggs, preferably eggs from pastured hens (these eggs offer better-quality protein). Egg yolk provides essential fats for our nervous systems as well as fat-soluble vitamins A and D.

It's all about eating real food! Real food contains cholesterol and fats that are healthy foods for you and your brain...and your children's brains, too.

## The Final Skinny:

Don't short-change your child's health potential by eating the SAD! SAD foods contain devitalized, substandard ingredients, especially when it comes to fats. Use what you've learned in this chapter and throughout this book to make healthier decisions for you and your family. Try making the recipes you'll find in Chapter 12.

You can also find out more about how to feed yourself and your family healthy, whole, **real** food in our book *The Guide to Healthy Eating*.

# (Endnotes)

1 http://www.naturalnews.com/035243_Russell_Blaylock_MSG_interview.html.

2 Is ADHD Caused By Insufficient Dietary Fat, Dr. Stephanie Seneff, senefff@csail.mit.edu, http://people.csail.mit.edu/seneff/adhd_low_fat_diet.html.

3 http://people.csail.mit.edu/seneff/adhd_low_fat_diet.html.

4 J Am Osteopath Assoc,111 (11): 610–4; 2011.

5 BMC Psychiatry, 10: 67; 2010.

6 http://www.cdc.gov/ncbddd/adhd/data.html.

# 11

# How to Cook With Fats and How to Store Them

**While fat is essential to our well-being**, it's important to do more than choose healthy, unrefined fats—we also need to make sure we're using the right kind of fats and oils for the right situations (high-heat cooking, medium-heat cooking and no-heat dishes). We also need to make our own dressings, spreads and other condiments with our healthy oils. In addition, we need to properly store fats and oils to preserve their health benefits. This is because different kinds of fat have varying degrees of stability—some hold up well to heat and some do not. That means some can be stored at room temperature, whereas others should be refrigerated.

Remember that saturated fat is solid at room temperature, while unsaturated fat is liquid. As mentioned in Chapter 3, there are three types of fat: saturated, monounsaturated, and polyunsaturated. The more unsaturated the oil is, the more vulnerable the oil is to oxidation and free radical formation. Heat, light, and oxygen all promote greater oxidation and the formation of free radicals. Remember from Chapter 3 that a free radical is a renegade molecule that disrupts healthy cell function and causes cell degeneration.

## Is Fat Good for Cooking/Baking?

Yes. Although many recipes tell you to omit fat or replace it with applesauce—or, even worse, to use low-fat or "heart-healthy" spreads which are inevitably made with refined, rancid vegetable oils—the key to healthy cooking and baking is really using the right fat for the job. Fat adds much needed nutrients and gives food a delicious taste as well. Fat also makes foods crispy and temptingly golden-brown when cooked and baked.

Saturated fat can handle high cooking temperatures thanks to its inherent stability. Not only will you **not** risk excess smoke (or a grease fire) when you cook with saturated fats, your fat won't sputter or spit out of the pan. That's less mess to clean up and fewer chances of getting burnt by flying oil. Common fats that are good for cooking with include butter, coconut oil, ghee, and tallow. You can also explore the use of other animal fats from pastured animals such as lard (pork fat), as well as duck, goose, or chicken fat for cooking or baking.

And then we have wonderful olive oil! It imparts a delicious flavor boost to salads, dips, and spreads. Skip those low-fat dressings and instead make your own with **extra-virgin** olive oil. (See the recipes in Chapter 12) Toss your salad with some fresh avocados, a free-range hard-boiled egg and a handful of nuts, and you have a flavorful, nutrient-rich, healthy meal. We generally recommend you stick to using olive oil for no heat situations such as salads or for occasional light cooking. Be sure to cook with it only at lower heat levels so you do not damage the wonderful properties of this amazing oil.

In addition to providing delicious flavor, fat gives food a creamy texture and makes meals more pleasing to eat. Considering that there's an endorphin (the "feel-good" chemical) release associated with fat, it's not surprising that fat enhances the pleasure of food. In short, fat triggers the release of satiety chemicals in the brain and makes you feel satisfied and full.

## What Is the Best Way to Cook With Fat and Oil?

As previously mentioned, unsaturated oils are susceptible to being damaged by light, heat, or oxygen. Knowing this makes it pretty obvious that it's not a good idea to cook with polyunsaturated oils at any temperature—they oxidize very quickly. Many of these are sold in cheap clear plastic containers and are already rancid before you even bring them home.

Monounsaturated oils can handle medium heat, but don't expose them to high temperatures. If you want to cook with high heat, opt for a saturated fat like butter, ghee, or coconut oil. Here's a quick breakdown of each type of fat, from the least saturated to the most saturated.

## Polyunsaturated Fat:

Since polyunsaturated fat is liquid at room temperature and stays liquid even when refrigerated, this type of fat is often referred to as an "oil" rather than a "fat." From a molecular perspective, polyunsaturated oils (corn, soy, canola) have a less-tightly-built structure than saturated fats do, meaning that polyunsaturated oils have multiple double bonds and unpaired electrons that make these delicate oils susceptible to damage when heated or processed. Exposure to light or oxygen can quickly create rancidity in polyunsaturated oils.

Oils containing high amounts of omega-6 fats (sunflower, soy, corn, safflower oils) should **not** be used for cooking purposes. These delicate oils are damaged by exposure to high or prolonged heat. The vast majority of the vegetable oils (again- sunflower, soy, corn, safflower) we see on grocery store shelves have already been severely damaged by the high-heat, high-chemical processing techniques that are used to refine inexpensive oils.

Oils rich in omega-3 fats are definitely not good for cooking with any heat. Omega-3 fats are particularly fragile—they are prone to forming free radicals when exposed to high heat, oxygen and even light. Omega-3 fats are even more fragile than omega-6 fats are. These nutritious oils—notably flaxseed oil—are great to drizzle onto cooked dishes after they've cooled down. They can also be used on cold items such as salads.

## Monounsaturated Fat:

Monounsaturated fats such as avocado or olive oil are liquid or soft at room temperature but become semi-solid when refrigerated. Monounsaturated oils like olive or avocado are not as stable as saturated fats are, but neither are they as unstable as polyunsaturated oils are. That begs the question "Are they good to cook with?"

Although you don't have to worry about creating trans fats or even much free radical damage when you use monounsaturated oils for cooking (assuming that you don't expose them to high heat), we don't suggest using your high-quality extra-virgin olive oil for cooking since that heat will start to damage the compounds in the oil. However, olive oil can be used for lower-temperature heat (under 250°F) and light sautéing. Better yet, use it for salad dressings, dips, and spreads.

If you are going to opt for nut and seed oils, be careful to choose only high-quality, cold-pressed/expeller-pressed versions that are packaged in opaque containers. These protected-from-light oils will retain all their nutrients and will not contain damaging free radicals or chemical residues. These oils are excellent for drizzling on salads.

## Saturated Fat:

Saturated fat is solid at room temperature, and its tightly packed molecular structure means that saturated fat is inherently stable. In other words, saturated fats are ideal fats for cooking. Saturated fats include coconut oil, palm oil, butter, ghee, and tallow. Heat does not damage these fats or create free radicals. And you've already learned from this book that saturated fat is not the cause of heart disease!

In summary, cooking with fats and oils depends primarily on how much you want to heat the fat or oil. Smoke point is an important consideration, because when a fat or oil exceeds its smoke point, it is not ideal to consume since it's begun to break down and free radicals have begun to form. In other words, if you see smoke emanating from the oil you are using, it is a sign the oil has broken down and oxidized. Avoid heating oils to their smoke points! Remember that the higher the smoke point a fat has, the more suitable that fat is for high-heat cooking.

Many refined oils boast higher smoke points, but that's no benefit—you're starting out with an inferior oil. Unprocessed polyunsaturated fats have low smoke points and are not suitable to use for cooking. Unprocessed monounsaturated fats have higher smoke points—they fall somewhere in the middle and can be used for low to medium heat.

Refer to the following tables for various fats and oils and their benefits and cooking uses.

**Table 16: Healthy Supplemental Oils:
NO HEAT**

| | |
|---|---|
| Cod Liver Oil* (never heat) | Supplemental oil rich in vitamins A and D; source of long-chain essential fatty acids EPA and DHA |
| Flaxseed Oil (never heat) | An essential fatty acid rich in omega-3 fats; use in smoothies, salad dressings, spreads or dips; drizzle on soups, cooked grains and cooked vegetables |
| High Vitamin Butter Oil* (never heat) | Source of Activator X—aids mineral utilization (synergistic with cod liver oil) |

**See resources in Appendix B for suggested Brands*

**Table 17: Healthy Cooking Oils:**

| | | |
|---|---|---|
| Butter, preferably from grass-fed cows (saturated fat) | Medium- to high-heat cooking; smoke point 350°F | Replaces margarine and is ideal for sautéing, baking, adding to vegetables or spreading liberally on bread |
| Coconut Oil (saturated fat) | High heat cooking; smoke point 350°F | For frying and higher-heat cooking; use with vegetables or as spread; use in cooking or baking; add to smoothies; add to popcorn |
| Extra-Virgin Olive Oil (monounsaturated fat) | Low- to medium-heat cooking; smoke point 375°F | For light sautéing; use in salad dressings or over vegetables; use in spreads, condiments and marinades |
| Ghee or Clarified Butter (saturated fat) | High heat cooking; smoke point 385°F | Replacement for casein-sensitive people; has a higher smoke point than butter does, so it's ideal for baking, high-heat cooking; use in dipping sauces or condiments |
| Lard (monounsaturated fat) | High-heat cooking; smoke point 370°F | Use in baking, especially pie crusts; use for frying and sautéing |

| | | |
|---|---|---|
| Palm Oil (saturated fat) | High-heat cooking; smoke point 440°F | Replaces shortening—use for baking, frying and making French fries |
| Peanut Oil (monounsaturated fat) | High-heat cooking; smoke point 385°F | Unrefined version is good for occasional stir-frying. |
| Sesame Oil | High-heat cooking; smoke point 350°F | Unrefined version is good for occasional stir-frying |
| Tallow (saturated fat) | High-heat cooking; smoke point 420°F | Frying,cooking eggs, sautéing |
| Corn, Soy, Canola, Cottonseed | | Avoid! Rancid, bleached, deodorized! |

## How Do I Purchase and Store Oils?

It is important to choose high-quality oils that have not been processed with high heat, chemicals, and pressures. Additionally, you might want to avoid oils produced from genetically modified crops. We suggest you look for organic oils that are expeller- or cold-pressed. These oils are your best options. But remember: you don't want to buy a cold-pressed oil and then go home and fry with it. That defeats the purpose since heat will accelerate the formation of free radicals and, therefore, turn the once-healthy oil into an unhealthy product. Basically, the more unrefined an oil is, the more gently we need to treat the oil.

When looking for good-quality oils, look for oils in dark, opaque containers. Opaque containers shield oil from light damage. Avoid oils packaged in clear plastic containers! And know that once opened, oxygen gets inside the container and can begin breaking down the oil. Fortunately, you can slow this process dramatically by refrigerating your oils once you've opened them.

Be extra careful with extra-fragile oils such as flaxseed and walnut oil. These should be packaged in dark, opaque (often glass) containers, and these oils should be immediately refrigerated when you get them home. Refrigerate them even before you open them.

When it comes to olive oil, choose extra-virgin olive oil that's packaged in dark glass containers. If you're going to use your olive oil within three to six months, you can store it in a cool, dark area (not above or next to the stove/oven!) to maximize the flavor and health benefits of the oil. If you're not going to use your olive oil quickly, store it in the refrigerator.

In the case of coconut oil, again try to find extra-virgin varieties. Coconut oil is a saturated fat, so it's shelf-stable and does not need to be refrigerated. Its stability also means that coconut oil can be packaged in clear glass containers. See Appendix B for resources for fats and oils.

## What About Salad Dressing?

We suggest that you not buy pre-made salad dressing. There is no better way to ruin a healthy salad than by putting an unhealthy salad dressing on it. Nearly all commercial brands are made with substandard, refined/rancid oils like soybean and canola. Making your own dressing is so simple. It's also less expensive than buying an entire bottle since you can make exactly as much as you need, plus your homemade dressing won't contain rancid vegetable oils, trans fats, or chemical additives. Delicious, nutritious dressing takes about one minute to make. Try the recipes in Chapter 12 or concoct your own creations!

## A Few Words About Storing Olive Oil

Since it's one of America's favorite oils, it's worth pointing out that extra-virgin olive oil is very easily damaged by light. Have you ever gone to a restaurant and seen olive oil sitting on your table in a clear glass bottle? This oil is more than likely rancid. Avoid it. Bring a small, discrete bottle of your own healthy olive oil to the restaurant.

In terms of storing your high-quality extra-virgin olive oil at home, either refrigerate it or keep it in a dark, cool cabinet away from the stove or any other source of heat or light. Heat, light or exposure to oxygen can cause the nutritional content of olive oil to rapidly deteriorate, especially its valuable vitamin E content.

## The Final Skinny:

Not all fats and oils are good for cooking. Heat, oxygen, and light can cause damaging molecular changes in oils, and some oils are better than others at resisting the stress of heat. Polyunsaturated oils and oils high in omega-3's in particular are fragile under heat, but monounsaturated oils are not as fragile. Saturated oils are the most stable of all and should be your go-to fat for higher heat cooking.

Keep in mind that proper packaging by the manufacturer and careful storage at home are important to preserve nutrients and prevent rancidity in oils. Heat, light, and oxygen are the most common damaging elements for oils. Be sure to buy cold-pressed or expeller pressed oils properly sealed in dark glass containers and refrigerate oils after opening them. In the case of olive oil, we suggest cold-pressed, extra-virgin found in dark glass containers.

# 12

# Recipes

BREAKFAST:

Cinnamon Waffles
Egg Sandwich
French Toast
Spinach Egg Bake
Veggie Quiche Cups

SMOOTHIES:

Avocado Almond Smoothie
Avocado Fruit Smoothie
Be Healthy! Smoothie
Blueberry Banana Smoothie
Chia Seed Smoothie
Piña Colada Smoothie

SPREADS:

Cinnamon Coconut Oil Spread
Honey Coconut Butter Spread
Strawberry Coconut Butter Spread

APPS AND DIPS:

Guacamole Dip
Hummus Dip
Pineapple Chipotle Salsa
Raw Grape Tomato Salsa
Spicy Guacamole with Cherry Tomatoes

Yogurt Fruit Dip
Yogurt Ranch Vegetable Dip
Zucchini Dip

## SOUPS:

Chicken Tortilla Soup
Grace's Greek Lemon Chicken Soup
Lentil Soup
Sweet Potato Soup
Thai Style Chicken Soup

## LUNCH AND DINNER ENTREES:

Cheese Quesadillas
Chicken & Vegetable Stew
Creamy Chicken and Basil
Crockpot Chili
Crockpot Coconut Chicken Curry
Juicy Hamburgers
Pineapple Salsa Salmon
Turkey Taco Salad
Wild Salmon with Pecan Crust

## SIDE DISHES:

Black-Eyed Pea Salad with Basil Dressing
Coconut Sweet Potato Puree
Coconut Green Beans
Healthy Sausage Stuffing

## SNACKS AND DESSERTS:

Apple Crisp

Baked Custard

Banana-Oat-Raisin Cookies

Coconut Cacao Bites

Nick's Nutty Fruit Cobbler

Peach Coconut Milk Ice Cream

## SALAD DRESSINGS:

Balsamic Dressing

Coconut Oil Dressing

Creamy Coconut Balsamic Dressing

Honey Mustard Dressing

Simple Greek-Style Dressing

Vinaigrette Dressing

Zesty Lime Vinaigrette

# BREAKFAST:

## Cinnamon Waffles

2 cups whole grain spelt flour or gluten-free flour mixture
1⅔ cups whole-milk plain organic yogurt or kefir
3 free-range eggs
1 tablespoon grass-fed butter or coconut oil, melted
1 tablespoon raw honey
1 teaspoon baking soda
1 teaspoon sea salt
1 teaspoon cinnamon
¼ teaspoon nutmeg
1–2 tablespoons filtered water
Grass-fed butter

**Servings:** 6–8 **Prep:** 10 minutes **Cook:** 15 minutes

Combine spelt flour with yogurt or kefir and let soak overnight. Blend in remaining ingredients, adding water to thin if necessary. Pour by spoonfuls onto a well greased (try coconut oil) waffle maker and heat through according to manufacturer instructions. Serve topped with butter.

***Other Serving Suggestions:*** *Top with Honey Coconut Butter, page 172, real maple syrup, fruit, or preserves.*

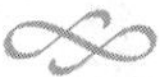

# Egg Sandwich

2 teaspoons coconut oil or tallow
1 free-range egg
1 piece sprouted whole-grain bread or gluten-free bread
1 tablespoon grass-fed butter (or more to taste)
1 tablespoon organic, cultured cream cheese (optional)
1 pinch sea salt

**Servings:** 1 **Prep:** 5 minutes **Cook:** 8 minutes

Heat pan over medium heat. Melt coconut oil or tallow and crack egg into pan. Cook egg 2–3 minutes until top of white has just begun to set. Flip and cook 1–2 more minutes ("over-easy" style egg). While egg is cooking, toast the bread. Spread toasted bread with butter and cream cheese and place cooked egg on top. Sprinkle with sea salt and serve.

***Serving Suggestions:*** *Serve with thinly sliced tomato.*

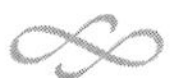

# French Toast

1 tablespoon coconut oil, grass-fed butter, or ghee
4 free-range eggs, lightly beaten
1 tablespoon heavy organic cream or coconut milk (full-fat)
1 teaspoon vanilla
½ teaspoon cinnamon
¼ teaspoon nutmeg
6 slices sprouted whole-grain bread
Grass-fed butter

**Servings:** 3–4 **Prep:** 10 minutes **Cook:** 10 minutes

Heat coconut oil, butter, or ghee in skillet over medium heat. Combine eggs, cream or coconut milk, vanilla, cinnamon and nutmeg in square dish. Dip bread into egg mixture to cover both sides. Cook in skillet until lightly browned on both sides. Serve topped with butter.

***Other Serving Suggestions:*** *Top with Honey Coconut Butter, page 172, Cinnamon Coconut Oil Spread, page 172, and/or maple syrup.*

***Storage Suggestion:*** *Make in large batches and separate with waxed paper before storing. Store them in the freezer for quick reheating in the toaster.*

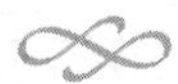

# Spinach Egg Bake

| | |
|---|---|
| 4 | free-range eggs |
| 2 | cups organic, heavy cream (preferably raw) |
| 2 | cups shredded raw cheese (e.g., raw-milk Gruyere) |
| ½-1 | cup chopped spinach |
| ½ | teaspoon sea salt |

**Servings:** 6–8 **Prep:** 10 minutes **Cook:** 30 minutes

Preheat oven to 425°F. Grease pie dish with butter or coconut oil and sprinkle the cheese to make the crust. Whisk together the eggs and cream. Blend in the spinach and sea salt. Pour mixture over the cheese in the pie dish. Bake 25–30 minutes or until lightly browned and slightly firm like custard.

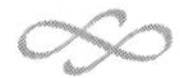

# Veggie Quiche Cups

1 tablespoon grass-fed butter, ghee, or tallow
⅓ cup diced red bell pepper
¼ cup diced onion
6 oz fresh baby spinach, chopped
5 free-range eggs, beaten
¾ cup shredded raw cheese (e.g., raw-milk Gruyere)
Sea salt and pepper to taste
Organic, full-fat sour cream

**Servings:** 4–6 **Prep:** 10 minutes **Cook:** 20 minutes

Preheat oven to 350ºF. Melt butter, ghee or tallow in pan and sauté pepper and onion until they start to soften. Add spinach and sauté until it wilts and liquid in the bottom of the pan evaporates; set aside to cool. Line a muffin tray with 9 baking cups. Mix beaten eggs, cooled vegetable mixture and shredded cheese. Season with sea salt and pepper. Fill muffin cups evenly and bake for 20 minutes or until cooked through. Serve with a side of sour cream.

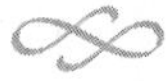

# SMOOTHIES:

## Avocado Almond Smoothie

1 avocado, ripe
1 apple
½ cup coconut milk (full-fat) or Amasai (see resources)
½ cup filtered water
2 tablespoons raw, organic almond butter
¼ teaspoon cinnamon (optional)
2 teaspoons raw honey or to taste (optional)

**Servings:** 2–4 **Prep:** 5 minutes **Blend:** 2 minutes

Add all ingredients to blender. Blend until smooth and serve. Add filtered water if necessary to desired consistency.

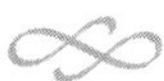

## Avocado Fruit Smoothie

½ avocado, ripe
1 cup frozen mangoes
½ cup frozen strawberries
½ cup filtered water
½ cup coconut milk (full-fat) or organic whole-milk yogurt
1–2 teaspoons raw honey (or to taste)

**Servings:** 1–2 **Prep:** 5 minutes **Blend:** 2 minutes

Add all ingredients to blender. Blend until smooth and serve. Add filtered water if necessary to desired consistency.

## Be Healthy! Smoothie

- ½ cup organic, whole milk yogurt, kefir, or Amasai (see resources)
- ½ cup filtered water
- 1 cup frozen fruit: blueberries, strawberries, raspberries, etc
- 1 tablespoon chia seeds
- 1 teaspoon cod liver oil (optional)
- 1 raw free-range egg yolk (optional)

**Servings:** 1–2 **Prep:** 5 minutes **Blend:** 2 minutes

Blend all ingredients until smooth and serve. Add filtered water if necessary to desired consistency.

***Serving Suggestions:*** *Add raw honey to taste and serve chilled.*

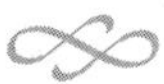

## Blueberry Banana Smoothie

- 1 cup frozen blueberries
- ½ banana, fresh or frozen
- ½ cup coconut milk (full-fat) or Amasai (see resources)
- ½ cup filtered water
- 2 teaspoons raw honey (optional)
- 1 raw free-range egg yolk (optional)

**Servings:** 1–2 **Prep:** 5 minutes **Blend:** 2 minutes

Blend all ingredients until smooth and serve. Add filtered water if necessary to desired consistency.

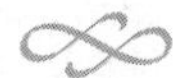

## Chia Seed Smoothie

1 cup coconut milk (full-fat) or Amasai (see resources)
1 cup frozen strawberries
1 banana, fresh or frozen
1 tablespoon chia seeds
2 teaspoons raw honey or to taste (optional)

**Servings:** 1–2 **Prep:** 5 minutes **Blend:** 2 minutes

Mix together in a blender until smooth and creamy. Add filtered water if necessary to desired consistency.

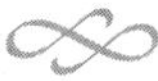

## Piña Colada Smoothie

1 frozen banana
1 cup coconut milk
1–2 teaspoons shredded coconut
¼ cup pineapple, chopped or crushed

**Servings:** 1–2 **Prep:** 5 minutes **Blend:** 2 minutes

Mix together in a blender until smooth and creamy. Add filtered water if necessary to desired consistency.

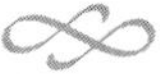

# SPREADS:

## Cinnamon Coconut Oil Spread

2 tablespoons coconut oil, softened
¼ teaspoon cinnamon
1 teaspoon raw honey

**Servings:** 3–4 **Prep:** 5 minutes

Beat oil, cinnamon and raw honey together until smooth. Can be stored covered on the counter or in the refrigerator.

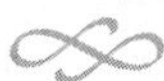

## Honey Coconut Butter Spread

2 teaspoons raw honey, melted
1 tablespoon coconut oil, softened
½ stick grass-fed butter, softened

**Servings:** 4 **Prep:** 5 minutes

Beat all ingredients together until smooth and creamy. Store covered in the refrigerator.

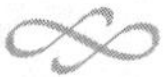

## Strawberry Coconut Butter Spread

- 2 teaspoons organic strawberry preserves (fruit-only jam; no sugar added!)
- ½ tablespoon coconut oil, softened
- ½ stick grass-fed butter, softened

**Servings:** 4 **Prep:** 5 minutes

Beat all ingredients together until smooth and creamy. Store covered in the refrigerator.

***Serving Suggestions for all spreads:*** *Spread on toast, Cinnamon Waffles, page 164, or French Toast, page 166.*

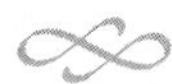

# APPS AND DIPS:

## Guacamole Dip

2 ripe avocados
2 tablespoons lemon
1 cup tomato, chopped
¼ cup onion, chopped
2 cloves garlic, minced
2 teaspoons sea salt
¼ teaspoon cayenne

**Servings:** 4–6 **Prep:** 10–15 minutes

Scoop avocados out of their shells and mash them in a bowl. Cover with lemon juice to prevent browning. Add remaining ingredients and mix well. Chill and serve.

***Serving Suggestions**: Great with blue chips or on salads.*

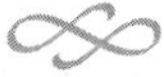

# Hummus Dip

2 cups garbanzo beans (canned or cooked)
2 cloves garlic, crushed
3 tablespoons tahini
½ cup lemon juice
1 tablespoon extra-virgin olive oil
1 teaspoon cold-pressed flax oil
1 teaspoon cumin
2 dashes cayenne (add to taste)
¼ teaspoon sea salt

**Servings:** 6 **Prep:** 15 minutes

Process cooked garbanzo beans in food processor until smooth. Add remaining ingredients and blend to desired consistency.

Note: To make smoother, add water or more olive oil.

***Serving Suggestion**: Put in bowl and pour 1 tablespoon olive oil over top, then sprinkle with paprika, Kalamata olives and/or parsley.*

*Note: For optimal results with non-canned beans (and for optimal digestion), we suggest you soak your beans overnight as follows before cooking: 1 cup beans, 2 cups filtered water and 2 tablespoons lemon juice. Rinse beans after soaking.*

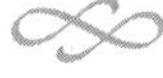

# Pineapple Chipotle Salsa

- 2 teaspoons coconut oil
- 3 cups pineapple, diced
- 1½ cups onion, chopped
- 1 cup seeded tomato, diced
- 2 cloves garlic, minced
- ½ cup pineapple juice
- 2 tablespoons coconut palm sugar
- 2 tablespoons apple cider vinegar
- 1 chipotle chile in adobo sauce, drained and minced
- 1 tablespoon adobo sauce (from drained chiles)
- ½ cup parsley, finely chopped
- 2 tablespoons fresh lime juice
- ½ teaspoon sea salt

**Servings:** 8 **Prep:** 10–15 minutes **Cook:** 10 minutes

Heat the coconut oil in a large skillet over medium-high heat. Add pineapple and onion and sauté 3–4 minutes or until lightly browned. Add tomato and garlic and sauté 2–3 minutes. Stir in pineapple juice, coconut palm sugar, vinegar, chile and adobo sauce. Cook 6 minutes, stirring occasionally. Remove from heat and stir in parsley, lime juice and salt.

***Serving Suggestions**: Serve warm over Salmon, page 194, or refrigerate and serve cool as a salsa dip.*

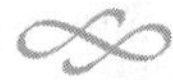

# Raw Grape Tomato Salsa

2 pints grape tomatoes
2 garlic cloves
½ cup each of parsley and cilantro
1 tablespoon apple cider vinegar
1 tablespoon extra-virgin olive oil
1 tablespoon lime juice
1 teaspoon each of cumin and sea salt
1 or 2 jalapenos, depending on your taste
2 green onions

**Servings:** 8 **Prep:** 10–15 minutes

Place everything except for the green onions in a food processor and pulse to chop. Hand-chop green onions and stir into salsa.

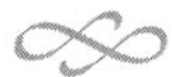

# Spicy Guacamole with Cherry Tomatoes

1 ripe avocado
1 tablespoon green chiles
2 tablespoons sweet onion, finely diced or grated
1 garlic clove, grated
¼ teaspoon cumin
Sea salt and black pepper to taste
1 lime, juiced
Approximately 20–24 cherry tomatoes
Cilantro for garnish (optional)

**Servings:** 8 **Prep:** 10–15 minutes

Mash avocado in a medium-sized bowl. Add the remaining ingredients (except for cherry tomatoes and cilantro) and blend thoroughly with a fork until mostly smooth. Prepare cherry tomatoes by cutting the tops off and scooping out the insides. Fill the tomatoes with the avocado mixture, and top with cilantro if desired. Serve cold.

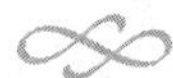

# Yogurt Fruit Dip

| | |
|---|---|
| 1½ | cups organic whole-milk yogurt (or Amasai – see resources) |
| ½ | cup organic cultured cream cheese |
| 2 | teaspoons vanilla |
| ½ | tablespoon maple syrup |

**Servings:** 8 **Prep:** 10–15 minutes

Place ingredients in a food processor and blend until smooth. Refrigerate before serving. Serve with fresh strawberries, grapes, pineapple, apples or other fruit you enjoy.

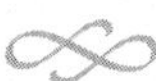

# Yogurt Ranch Vegetable Dip

| | |
|---|---|
| 1 | cup strained organic whole-milk yogurt (or Amasai – see resources) |
| 1 | teaspoon dill |
| ½ | teaspoon onion powder |
| ½ | teaspoon garlic powder |
| ½ | teaspoon parsley |

Sea salt and pepper to taste

**Servings:** 8 **Prep:** 10–15 minutes

Mix ingredients until well blended, adjust seasonings to taste. Refrigerate before serving. Serve with fresh chopped carrots, celery, bell peppers, broccoli, cucumbers or other vegetables you enjoy.

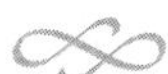

# Zucchini Dip

4 zucchini, shredded (unpeeled)
1 small onion, chopped
1 tablespoon sea salt
Filtered water to soak
1 cup organic, full-fat sour cream
2 teaspoons cumin
2 tablespoons lime juice
½ teaspoon fresh ground pepper

**Servings:** 8 **Prep:** 15 minutes

Combine zucchini, onion and sea salt in bowl. Cover with water and soak overnight. Squeeze out in a colander and mix in remaining ingredients. Chill and serve.

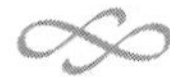

# SOUPS:

## Chicken Tortilla Soup

- 1 tablespoon coconut oil
- 1½ teaspoons cumin
- 1 teaspoon chili powder
- ½ teaspoon garlic powder
- ½ teaspoon sea salt
- 3 cloves garlic, minced
- ¼ cup diced green bell pepper
- ¼ cup diced red bell pepper
- 1 cup diced onion
- 10 ounce jar organic tomato sauce (in glass container)
- 48 ounces free-range chicken stock
- 3 tablespoons tomato paste
- 15 ounce can organic black beans, drained and rinsed
- 3 cups chopped cooked chicken meat

***Garnishes:*** *Organic corn or sprouted tortillas, sea salt, raw milk cheese, cilantro, and full-fat sour cream*

**Servings:** 6–8 **Prep:** 30 minutes **Cook:** 50 minutes

Heat oil in stock pan, add spices and cook stirring until fragrant. Add garlic, peppers and onion and cook until onion becomes translucent. Add remaining ingredients (except chicken), bring to a boil then reduce heat and simmer for 30 minutes. Adjust seasoning with salt and pepper. Stir in chicken.

Garnish: Organic corn or sprouted tortillas cut into strips and fried until crispy in coconut oil, sea salt while warm. Grated raw milk cheddar cheese tossed with chopped cilantro and sour cream.

# Grace's Greek Lemon Chicken Soup

6 cups free-range chicken stock
2 small carrots, peeled and small diced
6 free-range egg yolks
⅓ cup freshly squeezed lemon juice
1½ cups cooked chopped free-range chicken meat
1 cup raw organic long grain brown rice, cooked in 2½ cups water
2 tablespoons finely chopped parsley
Sea salt and pepper to taste

**Servings:** 6–8 **Prep:** 15–20 minutes **Cook:** 30 minutes

Heat chicken stock and carrots, simmer until carrots are tender. Whisk egg yolks and lemon juice together. While whisking, add 1 cup of hot chicken stock to the egg mixture in a slow stream, then return the egg mixture back to the pot. Simmer over medium heat, whisking periodically until mixture starts to thicken. Add chicken meat, cooked rice and parsley. Season with salt and pepper.

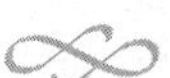

# Lentil Soup

½ cup coconut oil or ghee
2 onions, chopped
5 carrots, diced
4 stalks celery, chopped
5 cloves garlic, minced
1 bay leaf
2 teaspoons dried basil
6 cups lentils, washed and cleaned
1 can of crushed tomatoes (14.5 oz)
16 cups free-range chicken broth (or water)
2 cups chopped spinach
3 tablespoons balsamic vinegar
½ cup lemon juice
Sea salt and pepper to taste

***Garnish:*** *Raw shredded cheese*

**Servings:** 6–8 **Prep:** 15–20 minutes **Cook:** 75 minutes

In a large soup pot, heat oil over medium heat and add onions, carrots and celery. Cook and stir until onion is tender. Stir in garlic, bay leaf and basil and cook for 2 minutes. Stir in lentils, add water or broth and tomatoes. Bring to a boil. Reduce heat and simmer for at least 1 hour. When ready to serve, stir in spinach and cook until it wilts. Stir in vinegar, add lemon juice, and season to taste with salt and pepper. For a creamier soup, use an immersion blender, or blend only half the soup for a mixture of textures. Top with raw cheese and serve.

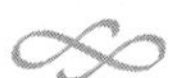

## Sweet Potato Soup

1 tablespoon unsalted grass-fed butter or ghee
1 Leek, white part only, halved, rinsed and thinly sliced
2 stalks celery, chopped
2 large sweet potatoes, peeled and cut into 2" pieces
4 cups chicken or vegetable broth
¼ cup toasted and chopped pecans (optional)
Sea salt and pepper

**Servings:** 6–8 **Prep:** 15–20 minutes **Cook:** 50 minutes

In a large saucepan over medium heat, melt the butter or ghee. Add the leek and celery and sauté until the leek is translucent, about 3 minutes. Add the potatoes and broth, raise the heat to high, and bring to a boil. Reduce the heat to low, cover, and simmer until the potatoes are tender, about 30 minutes. Using a food processor or blender, process the soup to a smooth puree. Return to the pan and reheat to serving temperature. Season to taste and garnish with pecans.

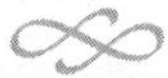

# Thai Style Chicken Soup

- 1 tablespoon coconut oil or ghee
- 3 shallots, chopped
- 2 tablespoons chopped cilantro
- 4 cups free-range chicken broth
- 28 ounces coconut milk (full-fat)
- 1 tablespoon raw honey
- 8 ounces crimini mushrooms, sliced
- 1 head broccoli, cut into florets
- 1 pound thinly sliced free-range chicken breast meat
- 2 teaspoons red curry paste
- 3 tablespoons lime juice
- 3 tablespoons fish sauce
- ½ cup chopped fresh cilantro
- 2 serrano chile peppers, thinly sliced
- ¼ cup chopped green onions
- 8 lime wedges

**Servings:** 6–8 **Prep:** 15–20 minutes **Cook:** 50 minutes

Heat the coconut oil in a large saucepan over medium heat. Cook the shallots with cilantro in the hot pan until the shallots have softened and become translucent, about 4 minutes. Add the chicken broth, coconut milk and raw honey. Bring to a simmer over medium-high heat. When the broth reaches a simmer, strain through a mesh strainer into a clean saucepan and discard the shallot and cilantro. Return the broth to a simmer. Stir in the mushrooms and broccoli and cook until the broccoli becomes tender, approximately 4 minutes. Add the chicken and cook until it is no longer pink, stirring constantly. Add the curry paste, lime juice, and fish sauce together in a small bowl to dissolve the curry paste. Mix the paste into the simmering soup. Ladle the soup into bowls and sprinkle with ½ cup cilantro, serrano peppers, green onions and lime wedges to serve.

# LUNCH AND DINNER ENTREES:

## Cheese Quesadillas

- 4 sprouted wheat tortillas
- 2 tablespoons grass-fed butter
- 2½ cups shredded raw cheese
- 1 tablespoon coconut oil

**Servings:** 2 **Prep:** 10 minutes **Cook:** 5 minutes

**Directions:**
Butter the outsides of the tortillas. Place cheese on non-buttered side of tortilla and make a sandwich with two tortillas, keeping buttered sides facing out. Cook in coconut oil at medium-high heat, flipping once, until both sides are lightly browned and cheese is melted in the middle.

***Serving Suggestions:*** *Add vegetables, beans, or meat to quesadilla.*

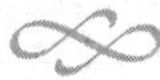

# Chicken & Vegetable Stew

1 pound boneless, skinless free-range chicken breasts
2 tablespoons coconut flour
1 teaspoon pepper
¼ teaspoon each thyme and dried parsley
1 tablespoon coconut oil
2–3 cloves garlic, minced
1 medium onion chopped
1 stalk celery, diced
1 cup free-range chicken broth
¼ cup fresh-pressed pineapple juice
1 cup carrots, chopped
12 oz can white beans, drained and rinsed
1 parsnip, cubed
2 bay leaves

**Servings:** 6–8 **Prep:** 15–20 minutes **Cook:** 40 minutes

Cut chicken into bite-sized cubes. In a bowl, combine flour, pepper, parsley and thyme. Dredge chicken cubes in mixture. Heat oil in a large pot on medium high. Add garlic, onion, celery and chicken cubes and sauté for 4–5 minutes. Turn heat down to medium and pour in stock and juice. Add carrots, beans, and parsnip and bay leaves and stir to combine. Cover and simmer on medium high until carrots and parsnips are soft, about 20 minutes. Uncover and cook for 5 minutes. Remove bay leaves and serve.

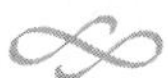

# Creamy Chicken and Basil

- 4 free-range chicken breasts
- 2 tablespoons coconut oil
- 1 cup organic, whole milk heavy cream preferably raw (or yogurt)
- 1 pinch sea salt
- 4 tablespoons grass-fed butter
- 2 tablespoons fresh basil, chopped finely
- 1 tablespoon sea salt
- 1 teaspoon black pepper
- 1 cup free-range chicken broth
- 2 tablespoons arrowroot
- 1 cup spinach, chopped

**Servings:** 4 **Prep:** 15 minutes **Cook:** 20 minutes

Sauté chicken in coconut oil about 4 minutes per side until almost fully cooked. Meanwhile, whip heavy cream and a pinch of sea salt with hand mixer until it begins to thicken. Pour whipped cream mixture along with butter, basil, salt and pepper into pan and bring to just under a boil. Combine broth with arrowroot and mix to dissolve. Pour slowly into cream mixture and stir slowly until thickened. Add chicken and spinach to pan and heat until spinach softens and chicken is cooked through.

***Serving Suggestions**: Serve over rice or quinoa.*

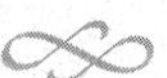

# Crockpot Chili

6 cups kidney beans (canned or cooked)
1 pound grass-fed ground beef
3 cups diced tomatoes
⅓ cup tomato paste
½ cup beef broth
½ onion, diced
2 teaspoons chili powder
3 teaspoons cumin
Sea salt, pepper, cayenne to taste
Raw cheese and full-fat sour cream

**Servings:** 4 **Prep:** 15 minutes **Slow Cook:** 5–6 hours

Drain and rinse beans before placing them into a crock pot. Brown beef, drain and add to crock pot. Add the rest of the ingredients and stir. Cover and cook in crock pot for 5–6 hours. Top with raw cheese and sour cream before serving.

***Other Serving Suggestions**: Serve with garnishes of cilantro, chopped onion, and/or jalapeno peppers.*

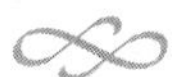

# Crockpot Coconut Chicken Curry

**Ingredients:**

1 tablespoon coconut oil
4 boneless skinless, free-range chicken breasts
3 medium potatoes, peeled and chopped
1 medium onion, sliced
14 ounces coconut milk (full-fat)
1 cup free-range chicken broth
1½ teaspoons curry powder
1 teaspoon hot pepper sauce
½ teaspoon sea salt
¼ to ½ teaspoon black pepper
10 ounces organic frozen peas
Hot cooked organic brown rice or quinoa

**Directions:**

1. Heat oil in large skillet over medium-high heat. Brown chicken on both sides. Place potatoes and onion in slow cooker. Top with chicken.
2. Combine coconut milk, broth, curry powder, pepper sauce, salt and pepper in medium bowl. Pour over chicken. Cover; cook on low 6 to 8 hours.
3. About 30 minutes before serving, add peas to slow cooker. Serve over hot cooked brown rice or quinoa.

**Servings:** 6–8 **Prep:** 15–20 minutes **Slow Cook:** 6–8 hours

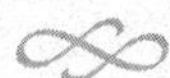

# Juicy Hamburgers

1 pound grass-fed ground beef
1 free-range organic egg
2 dashes naturally fermented or gluten free soy sauce
1 teaspoon each of sea salt and pepper
1 cup raw cheese, thinly sliced
4 sprouted, whole grain hamburger buns
Grass-fed butter

**Servings:** 4 **Prep:** 15 minutes **Cook:** 15 minutes

Combine beef, egg, soy sauce, sea salt and pepper in bowl and mash together until blended. Form into 4 hamburgers and grill to desired temperature. Top with raw cheese and let melt while still over heat. Toast or grill sprouted, whole grain hamburger buns with butter on them, add burgers and serve.

***Serving Suggestions**: Serve with ketchup, mustard, lettuce, tomato, onion, and/or guacamole, page 174.*

***Storage Suggestion:** Make in large batches without adding the cheese and freeze in preformed patties separated by waxed paper. For a quick meal, just remove from freezer and put on the grill!*

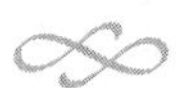

# Pineapple Salsa Salmon

1 tablespoon coconut oil
1 tablespoon grass-fed butter
2 wedges of lemon (juiced)
2 cloves garlic, crushed
1 pound wild salmon
1 recipe Pineapple Chipotle Salsa (see page 176)

**Servings:** 4 **Prep:** 10 minutes **Cook:** 20 minutes

Preheat oven to 350F. Combine coconut oil, butter, lemon, and garlic in small bowl. Spread mixture over salmon and then bake for 20 minutes, or to desired appearance. Top salmon with Pineapple Chipotle Salsa, page 176.

***Serving Suggestions**: Serve with a side of cream or sour cream.*

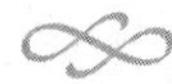

# Turkey Taco Salad

- 1 pound free-range ground turkey (or use grass-fed ground beef)
- 2 tablespoons grass-fed butter, ghee, or lard
- 2 tablespoons tomato paste
- 2–3 teaspoons chili powder
- 1½ teaspoons ground cumin
- ¼ teaspoon garlic powder
- ¼ teaspoon onion powder
- ¼ teaspoon paprika
- 1 teaspoon sea salt
- ½ teaspoon black pepper
- ½ cup chicken broth (or water)

**Servings:** 4 **Prep:** 10 minutes **Cook:** 25 minutes

Brown the turkey in a butter, ghee, or lard over medium-high heat. Drain meat and put back in skillet with all of the spices and broth. Simmer about 15 minutes, stirring occasionally.

***Serving Suggestions***: *Serve over lettuce with shredded raw cheese, tomatoes, black olives, black beans, sour cream or yogurt, and crumbled tortilla chips (optional). Great with Guacamole, page 174 or Spicy Guac, Page 178.*

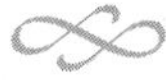

# Wild Salmon with Pecan Crust

2 tablespoons finely chopped fresh basil leaves
1 ½ tablespoons Dijon mustard
¼ teaspoon kosher salt
⅛ teaspoon black pepper
2 oz dry white wine
4 tablespoons fresh lemon juice
4 wild salmon fillets
2–4 tablespoons grass-fed butter or ghee
½ cup chopped raw pecans

**Directions:**
Preheat oven to 400°F. In a small bowl, mix together the basil, mustard, salt, pepper, white wine and lemon juice. Spread the mixture over the salmon, covering on all sides. Arrange salmon fillets in a shallow baking pan or sheet. Be sure to leave enough room between each one so they bake evenly. Mix the butter or ghee and pecans together, then spoon even amounts over each fillet, spreading out slightly to cover the top of the fillets. Place salmon in the preheated oven and cook for about 15 to 20 minutes. Check to ensure it is cooked through—when flaked apart with a fork, the salmon should be opaque. Serve hot.

**Servings:** 6–8 **Prep:** 15–20 minutes **Cook:** 20 minutes

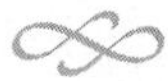

# SIDE DISHES:

## Black-Eyed Pea Salad with Basil Dressing

**Dressing:**

2 tablespoons raw apple cider vinegar

1 tablespoon plus 1 teaspoon chopped fresh basil, or ½ teaspoon dried

2 medium cloves of garlic, crushed

½ teaspoon coconut palm sugar

Sea salt and pepper

½ cup extra-virgin olive oil

Whisk all ingredients together.

**Combine dressing with:**

3 cups canned or cooked black-eyed peas (two 15 oz. cans, drained)

¼ teaspoon sea salt

½ cup each of finely chopped onion and celery

1 small red bell pepper, seeded and finely chopped

Refrigerate overnight or at least two hours.

**Servings:** 6–8 **Prep:** 15–20 minutes

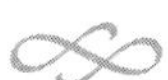

# Coconut Sweet Potato Puree

2 large sweet potatoes
⅔ cup coconut milk
2 teaspoons cinnamon
2 tablespoons vanilla extract
2 teaspoons maple syrup (or to taste)
½ teaspoon sea salt

*Garnish: organic, heavy cream and grass-fed butter*

**Servings:** 4 **Prep:** 10 minutes **Cook:** 60 minutes

Preheat oven to 400°F. Cut sweet potatoes in half and bake in center of oven for 1 hour or until tender when pierced with a fork. While baking, warm the coconut milk and cinnamon in a small sauce pan. Remove potatoes from oven and scoop flesh into a food processor. Process potatoes until they are smooth. Add vanilla, maple syrup, sea salt, cream, and butter and then process again. Put into a bowl and fold in the coconut milk and cinnamon mixture. Serve warm topped with heavy cream and butter.

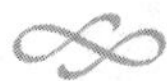

# Coconut Green Beans

- 1 tablespoon coconut oil
- ½ cup onion, chopped
- 2 tablespoons water
- 2 cloves garlic, minced
- 1 pound green beans, ends removed
- 1½ cups tomato, diced
- ¾ cup coconut milk (full-fat)
- ½ teaspoon sea salt

**Servings:** 4–6 **Prep:** 10 minutes **Cook:** 20 minutes

Sauté onion in coconut oil over medium-high heat for about 3–5 minutes. Add water, garlic and green beans. Stir fry for 8 to 10 minutes or until desired texture is reached. Add tomatoes, coconut milk and sea salt and heat through.

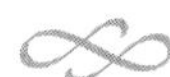

## Healthy Sausage Stuffing

1 pound turkey sausage, nitrite-and nitrate-free
2 tablespoons grass-fed butter, ghee, or lard
¼ cup finely chopped celery
¼ cup finely chopped onion
2 eggs
2 cups chopped cauliflower (bite-size)
½ cup chopped yellow squash (bite-size)
½ cup freshly grated Parmesan
1 tablespoon chopped fresh parsley
3 tablespoons chopped fresh sage
3 tablespoons chopped fresh thyme
1 garlic clove, grated
¼ teaspoon sea salt
⅛ teaspoon black pepper
Grass-fed butter (optional)

**Servings:** 6–8 **Prep:** 15–20 minutes **Cook:** 50 minutes

Preheat oven to 350ºF. If necessary, remove casing from sausage and break into small bits. Cook sausage in butter, ghee, or lard over medium heat. Add the celery and cook, stirring often, until the celery starts to get soft. Add onion and cook, stirring often, until the onion gets soft. Continue cooking, stirring often, until the sausage is completely cooked. Meanwhile, in a separate large bowl, beat the eggs. Add the cooked sausage mixture to the bowl, mix eggs into meat, then add remaining ingredients and mix together until completely blended. Place mixture into a 9 × 12 casserole dish, cover, and put in preheated oven. Bake 30 to 35 minutes. If stuffing is still too moist, uncover and continue cooking for 5 to 10 minutes more or until edges start to brown. Top with butter before serving.

# SNACKS AND DESSERTS

*Snacks and desserts are best made at home with the highest-quality ingredients you can find. Be sure to add some good-quality fats to balance the effect sweeteners have on your blood sugar. When it comes to nuts, buying raw nuts is optimal; also, soaking and dehydrating the nuts is ideal since doing so greatly aids their digestibility.*

## Apple Crisp

5–6 apples, cored and peeled
2 tablespoons maple syrup
2 teaspoons vanilla
1 teaspoon cinnamon
½ teaspoon sea salt
¼ teaspoon nutmeg
1 cup rolled oats
⅓ cup coconut palm sugar or Sucanat,™ whole cane sugar
½ cup grass-fed butter, not melted

**Servings:** 6 **Prep:** 15–20 minutes **Cook:** 30–33 minutes

Preheat oven to 400ºF. Put apples in 8 × 8 Pyrex dish and set aside. In small bowl, combine maple syrup, vanilla, cinnamon, salt and nutmeg. Pour over apples and gently toss until coated. Mix oats and coconut palm sugar or Sucanat™. Cut butter into the oat mixture. Sprinkle over the top of the apples. Bake on the bottom rack for 25–30 minutes or until apples are tender and bubbly. Move apple crisp to middle rack of oven and broil for 2–3 minutes or until top is lightly brown and crisp on top. Great served with homemade whipped cream on top!

# Baked Custard

| | |
|---|---|
| ¾ | cup organic, heavy cream |
| ⅛ | teaspoon sea salt |
| ¾ | cup coconut milk |
| 2 | free-range eggs, beaten |
| 2 | free-range egg yolks, beaten |
| 3 | tablespoons coconut palm sugar |
| 2 | teaspoons vanilla |

**Servings:** 6 **Prep:** 15 minutes **Cook:** 35 minutes

Preheat oven to 350°F. Mix cream with sea salt until slightly thick in food processor, about 2–3 minutes. Add the rest of the ingredients and process until smooth. Pour into 6 small ramekins and place them into a 9 × 13 inch dish. Fill dish halfway up the sides with water to create a bath for the ramekins. Bake for 35 minutes or until firm and lightly browned on top.

***Serving Suggestions**: For variation, serve with berries on top.*

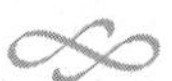

# Banana-Oat-Raisin Cookies

| | |
|---|---|
| ½ | cup oat flour |
| ½ | cup coconut flour |
| ½ | cup rolled oats |
| 1 | teaspoon baking soda |
| 1 | teaspoon cinnamon |
| ½ | teaspoon sea salt |
| ¾ | cup coconut palm sugar or Sucanat™, raw cane sugar |
| ½ | cup coconut oil or ghee |
| 1 | very ripe banana, mashed |
| 2 | eggs |
| 2 | teaspoons vanilla |
| ½ | cup raisins |

**Servings:** 12 **Prep:** 15 minutes **Cook:** 12–14 minutes

Preheat oven to 325ºF. In a medium bowl, mix together flours, oats, baking soda, salt and cinnamon. In a large bowl, cream the coconut palm sugar or Sucanat™ with the coconut/ghee. Add the banana eggs, and vanilla until blended. Slowly add flour mixture into banana mixture and stir until well combined. Add raisins or other optional items if desired and stir. Refrigerate 30 minutes. Drop by rounded spoonfuls onto lightly greased cookie sheet. Bake for 5 minutes and then push cookies down gently with a fork. Continue baking another 7 to 9 minutes or until lightly browned.

**Variation:** *Substitute chocolate chips and/or walnuts for raisins*

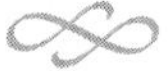

# Coconut Cacao Bites

- ⅓ cup raw honey
- 2 tablespoons coconut oil
- 3 tablespoons cacao powder
- ½ teaspoon cinnamon
- ¼ cup raw almond butter
- ½ cup rolled oats
- ¼ cup coconut flour
- 1 teaspoon vanilla extract

**Servings:** 12 **Prep:** 5 minutes **Cook:** 5 minutes

In a saucepan over medium heat, combine honey, coconut oil, cacao powder and cinnamon. Stir continuously until chocolate syrup-like texture. Remove from heat and add remaining ingredients. Stir until completely combined. Drop by the spoonful on waxed paper and chill approximately 45 minutes or until firm and chewy.

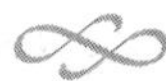

# Nick's Nutty Fruit Cobbler

- 3 cups fresh or frozen, thawed blueberries (or other fruit)
- ¼ cup lemon juice
- ⅔ cup coconut palm sugar
- 1½ cups raw pecans or other raw nuts
- ¾ teaspoon ground cinnamon
- 1 dash of sea salt
- 1 stick grass-fed butter, cold and chopped into pieces

**Servings:** 6 **Prep:** 10 minutes **Cook:** 25 minutes

Preheat oven to 350°F. Place berries in 8 × 8 inch baking dish and sprinkle with lemon juice. In a food processor, combine coconut palm sugar, nuts, cinnamon and salt. Add butter pieces to food processor and pulse until mixture resembles coarse crumbs. Sprinkle nut mixture over berries and bake for 20–25 minutes or until topping is golden brown and berries are tender.

***Serving Suggestions****: Serve warm or cold. A little fresh organic cream is a wonderful accompaniment!*

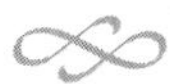

## Peach Coconut Milk Ice Cream

2 cups coconut milk
2 cups peaches, frozen
½ cup maple syrup
2 teaspoons vanilla
1 pinch sea salt

**Servings:** 4–6 **Prep:** 10 minutes

Put all ingredients in blender and blend until smooth. Pour in ice cream machine and freeze according to the machine's instructions.

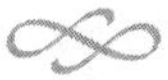

# SALAD DRESSINGS

*You can make your own salad dressing using the finest ingredients for about the same cost as an average bottle of dressing...and your homemade dressings* ***won't*** *contain rancid vegetable oils, trans fats or additives! With a little practice, it takes no more than a couple of minutes to produce a delicious dressing for your salad. Try the following recipes or concoct your own creations!*

## Balsamic Dressing

- 2 tablespoons aged balsamic vinegar
- 1 teaspoon Dijon mustard
- ½ teaspoon sea salt
- 1 clove garlic, minced
- ¼ cup extra virgin olive oil
- 1 teaspoon cold-pressed flax oil

**Servings:** 4 **Prep:** 10 minutes

Combine balsamic, mustard, salt and garlic in food processor. While processing, add olive oil in slow stream and then the flax oil. Refrigerate before serving.

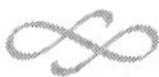

## Coconut Oil Dressing

¼ cup apple cider vinegar
¼ teaspoon sea salt
⅛ teaspoon white pepper
⅓ cup extra virgin olive oil
⅓ cup extra virgin coconut oil, melted

**Servings:** 4 **Prep:** 10 minutes

Combine apple cider vinegar, salt and pepper in a food processor. While processing, add two the oils. Serve.

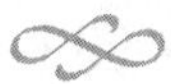

## Creamy Coconut Balsamic Dressing

⅛ cup coconut milk (full-fat)
1½ tablespoons aged balsamic vinegar
1 teaspoon Dijon mustard
½ teaspoon dried basil
¼ teaspoon sea salt
¼ cup extra-virgin olive oil
2 teaspoons cold-pressed flax oil

**Servings:** 4 **Prep:** 10 minutes

Combine coconut milk, balsamic, mustard, basil and salt in food processor. While processing, add olive oil in slow stream and then the flax oil. Refrigerate before serving.

# Honey Mustard Dressing

¼ cup lemon juice
2 tablespoons Dijon mustard
2 tablespoons raw honey
1 clove garlic, minced
1 dash cayenne pepper
½ cup extra virgin olive oil
2 teaspoons cold-pressed flax oil

**Servings:** 4 **Prep:** 10 minutes

Combine lemon juice, mustard, honey, garlic and cayenne pepper in food processor. While processing, add olive oil in slow stream and then the flax oil. Refrigerate before serving.

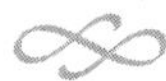

# Simple Greek-Style Dressing

½ cup lemon juice
2 cloves garlic
1 tablespoon dried oregano
1 cup olive oil
1 teaspoon cold-pressed flax oil
Sea salt and pepper

**Servings:** 4 **Prep:** 10 minutes

Combine lemon juice, garlic and oregano in food processor. While processing, add olive oil in slow stream and then the flax oil. Add sea salt and pepper to taste. Refrigerate before serving.

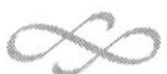

## Vinaigrette Dressing

½ cup apple cider vinegar
½ teaspoon raw honey
½ teaspoon mustard
½ teaspoon oregano
½ cup extra virgin olive oil
1 clove garlic, quartered
Sea salt and pepper to taste

**Servings:** 4 **Prep:** 10 minutes

Combine apple cider vinegar, raw honey, mustard and oregano in food processor. While processing, add olive oil in slow stream. Add salt and pepper to taste. Add garlic and refrigerate before serving. It is best to make several hours ahead of time so the garlic will flavor the dressing better. You may leave the garlic in or remove it if you want milder dressing.

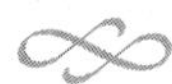

## Zesty Lime Vinaigrette

2 tablespoons soy sauce (naturally fermented or gluten-free)

⅓ cup lime juice

½ tablespoon raw honey

1 dash cayenne

1 cup extra virgin olive oil

Sea salt to taste

**Servings:** 4 **Prep:** 10 minutes

Combine soy sauce, lime, honey and cayenne in food processor. While processing, add olive oil in slow stream. Season with sea salt to taste. Refrigerate before serving.

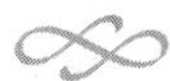

# Know Your Fats

# Quick Reference Guide

*Get a handy PDF version of this guide at www.sherylshenefelt.com under resources*

Fat is a macronutrient that is crucial to the proper functioning of our bodies. It plays many important roles, including being our main source of energy.

Fats are made up of individual fatty acid molecules which join together to make chains. These chains vary in length (short-, medium- or long-chain), and each type of fat offers different benefits. The structure of fat also determines whether a particular fat is solid or liquid at room temperature.

For years, we have been taught that fat should be avoided at all costs, but this is just not true. We need fats—the good fats—to live. Here is a brief summary of the good, the bad, and the ugly types of fat that we discuss in this book.

## THE GOOD FATS

Good fats are fats that have not been hydrogenated, manufactured with high temperatures or otherwise damaged in processing. Good fats include a variety of saturated, monounsaturated, and polyunsaturated fats. We suggest you include these fats regularly in your diet!

Our bodies use good fats (and cholesterol) to maintain healthy cells. Good fats also support healthy immune and hormonal systems. In this book we show you why—contrary to popular belief—healthy saturated fats actually fall into the **good** category when eaten with a balanced and varied diet. Good fats include items like butter, coconut oil, ghee, olive oil, avocado, nuts and seeds, and even animal fats like lard and tallow.

## THE BAD FATS

The bad fats include processed, heated, deodorized and/or bleached vegetable oils and rancid fats. We suggest you avoid these bad fats.

Examples include vegetable oils like corn, soy, canola, sunflower, safflower, and cottonseed oils. Any polyunsaturated oils that have been exposed to heat, light or oxygen in manufacturing should be avoided.

## THE UGLY FATS

Ugly fats include hydrogenated or partially hydrogenated oils and trans fats. These ugly fats are often found in margarine and spreads as well as many baked goods and processed foods. Vegetable oils that have gone through the interesterification process are even uglier than trans fats are. These altered fats have no place in the diet or in our food supply! Ugly fats offer no nutritional value and have been linked to the rises in obesity, metabolic syndrome, heart disease, and cancer.

## SUMMARY OF GOOD FATS TO INCLUDE

- Avocado
- Butter (grass-fed)
- Chia seeds
- Coconut oil
- Coconut milk
- Cod liver oil
- Duck, chicken, and goose fat
- Flax oil and seeds
- Ghee (clarified butter)
- Lard
- Nuts and seeds
- Nut and Seed Oils (Expeller/Cold-Pressed)
- Olive oil (extra-virgin)
- Palm oil
- Pastured/grass-fed meats
- Sesame oil (expeller pressed)
- Tallow

## SUMMARY OF BAD AND UGLY FATS TO AVOID

- Canola oil
- Corn oil
- Soybean oil
- "Vegetable" oil
- Peanut oil (refined)
- Sunflower oil
- Safflower oil
- Cottonseed oil
- Grapeseed oil
- Margarine
- Shortening
- I Can't Believe It's Not Butter (You better believe it!)
- Smart Balance (Not a smart idea!)
- Any fake butter or vegetable oil products

# Coconut Oil

# Quick Reference Guide

*Get a handy PDF version of this guide at www.sherylshenefelt.com under resources*

Coconut oil is a healthy fat great for cooking and baking, as well as for its ability to help with thyroid, hormonal, and weight issues. Coconut oil is also known for its lauric acid content and its immune enhancing properties. Lauric acid has been shown in various scientific studies to contain bacterial and anti-viral properties.

## Health Qualities of Coconut Oil:

- ☑ Anti-candida
- ☑ Boost your daily energy and support your thyroid function
- ☑ Burns quickly for energy—medium-chain fats
- ☑ Healthy form of saturated fat
- ☑ Immune booster—contains lauric and capric acid
- ☑ Increases metabolism
- ☑ No refrigeration necessary
- ☑ Thyroid support
- ☑ Very stable oil—withstands heat, good for cooking

## Seven Reasons to Use Coconut Oil:

1. Boost your daily energy and support thyroid function
2. Help you lose weight or maintain your weight
3. Improve conditions in those with diabetes and chronic fatigue
4. Improve Crohn's, IBS and other digestive disorders
5. Support your immune system and help prevent illnesses due to powerful antibacterial, antiviral, and antifungal agents
6. Reduce the risk of heart disease
7. Rejuvenate hair, skin, and for preventing wrinkles

## Tips to Implement Coconut Oil in Your Diet:

- ☑ Use as replacement for shortening, margarine, and all processed oils (soy, corn, canola, etc.)

- ☑ Use for baking brownies, cakes, cookies, muffins, etc.
- ☑ Use to fry foods or sauté vegetables, meats, eggs, etc.
- ☑ Use on popcorn along with some Celtic sea salt for a great snack!
- ☑ Spread on bread (try ½ butter and ½ coconut oil mixed together)
- ☑ Take as a supplement—stir 1–2 Tbsp into warm water or tea and drink before meals; this is especially great for weight loss and combating candida
- ☑ Mix into soups or stews
- ☑ Spread on face and body as a great skin moisturizer
- ☑ Rub it into your hair and scalp for healthy, shiny hair and to reduce dry scalp

## Forms of Coconut to Explore in Your Diet:

- ☑ Coconut cream
- ☑ Coconut milk
- ☑ Coconut vinegar
- ☑ Coconut palm sugar
- ☑ Coconut water
- ☑ Dried unsweetened coconut flakes
- ☑ Freeze-dried coconut

## Use for Coconut Items in Your Diet:

- ☑ Add coconut milk or cream to soups, smoothies, shakes, ice cream or other desserts (10 ounces of coconut milk yields about 3.5 ounces of coconut oil)
- ☑ Add coconut milk, cream, or flakes to oatmeal
- ☑ Add coconut flakes to trail mix or sprinkle into yogurt
- ☑ Use coconut palm sugar instead of white sugar in your recipes
- ☑ Drink coconut water as a sports drink to replace electrolytes after a workout
- ☑ Use coconut vinegar in salad dressings or spreads

# 5 Steps to Optimal Health

# With Good Fats

*Get a handy PDF version of this guide at www.sherylshenefelt.com under resources*

## STEP 1

**Avoid** low- and non-fat items such as milk, yogurt, cheese and other dairy products. Avoid low- and non-fat processed foods.

**Use** full-fat dairy products from grass-fed/pastured animals and from farmers you trust (preferably organic and raw or low-heat pasteurized) Find sources at www.localharvest.org.

## STEP 2

**Avoid** margarine and hydrogenated oils and spreads.

**Use** butter or ghee for cooking and spread them liberally on vegetables, sprouted breads, etc.

## STEP 3

**Avoid** canola and other processed vegetable oils such as soy, corn, cottonseed, safflower or sunflower oil.

**Use** traditional fats such as coconut oil, palm oil, lard, tallow or olive oil in place of vegetable oils.

## STEP 4

**Avoid** store-bought dressing with additives, flavorings and hydrogenated or processed oils.

**Use** your own salad dressings—explore olive oil, cold-pressed sesame oil or cold-pressed flax oil!

## STEP 5

**Avoid** snacks and processed foods with hydrogenated oils, trans fats or interesterified oils. Always read ingredient labels on peanut butter, chips and most processed foods in a box, bag or package. Also be wary of baked goods such as cookies, cakes, muffins and crackers.

**Use** real-food ingredients and prepare or bake snacks and desserts at home using real fats like butter and coconut oil! While you're at it, replace white sugar with stevia, raw honey or coconut palm sugar.

# Appendix A: Glycemic Index of Carbohydrates

The glycemic index is a measure of the speed of entry of carbohydrates into the bloodstream. Since carbohydrates cause blood sugar to rise, resulting in an elevated insulin level, it is recommended to limit the foods with the highest glycemic index and to eat foods with the lowest glycemic index (i.e., those with an index <50%). Also, remember that consuming good fats along with carbohydrate-rich foods helps reduce the glycemic impact on the body and is just one of the many great reasons to include those good fats with every meal!

**High glycemic index, greater than 100% ('Bad' carbohydrates)**

*Grain-Based Foods*

- Puffed rice
- Corn flakes
- Puffed wheat
- Millet
- Instant rice
- Instant potato
- Microwaved potato
- French bread

*Simple Sugars*

- Maltose
- Glucose

*Snacks*

- Tofu ice cream
- Puffed-rice cakes

**Glycemic Index Standard = 100%**

- White Bread

**Glycemic Index between 80 and 100%**

*Grain-based foods*

- Grape-Nuts
- Whole wheat bread
- Rolled oats
- Oat bran
- Instant mashed potatoes
- White rice
- Brown rice
- Muesli
- Shredded wheat

*Vegetables*

- Carrots
- Parsnips
- Corn

*Fruits*

- Banana
- Raisins
- Apricots
- Papaya
- Mango

*Snacks*

- Ice cream (low fat)
- Corn chips
- Rye crisps

**Glycemic index between 50 and 80%**

*Grain-based foods*

- Spaghetti (white)
- Spaghetti (whole wheat)
- Pasta, other
- Pumpernickel bread
- Fruits
- Kiwi
- Orange
- Orange juice

*Vegetables*

- Beets
- Peas
- Sweet potato
- Pinto beans
- Garbanzo beans
- Kidney beans (canned)
- Baked beans
- Navy beans

*Simple sugars*

- Lactose
- Sucrose

**Glycemic index between 30 and 50%**

*Grain based foods*

- Barley
- Oatmeal (slow cooking)
- Whole grain bread

*Fruits*

- Apple
- Apple juice
- Applesauce
- Grapes
- Peaches
- Pears

*Vegetables*

- Kidney beans (fresh)
- Black-eyed peas
- Chick-peas
- Lima beans
- Tomato soup
- Dairy Products
- Ice cream (high fat)
- Milk
- Yogurt

**Glycemic index less than 30% ('Good' carbohydrates)**

*Fruits*

- Cherries
- Plums
- Grapefruit

*Vegetables*

- Green vegetables
- Lentils

*Simple sugars*

- Fructose
- Nuts

# Appendix B: Other Resources

These are just a few of the resources the authors use regularly and have referred to in this book. Of course, there are many great options available and we encourage the reader to research and find the highest quality fats, supplements, and superfoods possible. A great place to find trustworthy resources is in the Shopping Guide which can be purchased from The Weston A. Price Foundation at www.westonaprice.org.

**Butter –**

Grass-fed from a local farmer is optimal—find one near you at www.localharvest.org.
At the store some good options include: Kalona SuperNatural organic butter, Kerrygold butter, Organic Valley Pastured Butter.

**Coconut Oil –**

Omega Nutrition www.omeganutrition.com
Tropical Traditions www.tropicaltradtions.com
Wilderness Family Naturals www.wildernessfamilynaturals.com

**Cod Liver Oil and High Vitamin Butter Oil –**

Raw, Extra Virgin Cod Liver Oil www.corganic.com/evclo
Radiant Life www.4radiantlife.com

**Amasai—**

Cultured dairy with over 30 probiotics made from A2 dairy cows that are 100% grass-fed and organic. Available online at: www.sherylshenefelt.com/products

**Total Liver Cleanse (TLC)—**

Liver detoxing product created by Dr. Brownstein and his partners at Center For Holistic Medicine. Available online at: store.centerforholisticmedicine.com

# About the Authors

## David Brownstein, M.D.

David Brownstein, M.D. is a Board-Certified family physician who utilizes the best of conventional and alternative therapies. He is the Medical Director for the Center for Holistic Medicine in West Bloomfield, MI. He is a graduate of the University of Michigan and Wayne State University School of Medicine. Dr. Brownstein is a member of the American Academy of Family Physicians and the American College for the Advancement in Medicine. He is the father of two beautiful girls, Hailey and Jessica and is a retired soccer coach. Dr. Brownstein has lectured internationally about his success using natural items. Dr. Brownstein has authored thirteen books: *Iodine: Why You Need It, Why You Can't Live Without It, 5th Edition; Vitamin B12 for Health; Drugs That Don't Work and Natural Therapies That Do, 2nd Edition; The Miracle of Natural Hormones 3rd Edition; Overcoming Thyroid Disorders 3rd Edition; Overcoming Arthritis; Salt Your Way to Health, 2nd Edition; The Guide To Healthy Eating, 2nd Edition; The Guide to a Gluten-Free Diet, 2nd Edition; The Guide to a Dairy-Free Diet; The Soy Deception,* and his newest books *The Skinny on Fats* and *The Statin Disaster.*

Dr. Brownstein is the author of *Dr. Brownstein's Natural Way to Health Monthly Newsletter*. His weekly blog can be accessed on his website at www.drbrownstein.com.

Dr. Brownstein's office is located at:
Center for Holistic Medicine
5821 W. Maple Rd.
Ste. 192
West Bloomfield, MI 48322
248.851.1600

**www.drbrownstein.com**
**www.centerforholisticmedicine.com**

Join in the conversations with Dr. Brownstein at:
**Facebook:** www.facebook.com/drdavidbrownstein
**Twitter:** www.twitter.com/drbrownstein
**YouTube:** www.youtube.com/user/drdavidbrownstein

## Sheryl Shenefelt, C.N., CMTA

Sheryl Shenefelt is a Certified Nutritionist and co-author of 5 books including: *The Guide to Healthy Eating, 2nd Edition; The Guide to a Gluten-Free Diet, 2nd Edition; The Guide to a Dairy-Free Diet; The Soy Deception;* and *The Skinny on Fats* with Dr. Brownstein. As a nutritional consultant and holistic health coach, Sheryl is dedicated to serving the nutritional, lifestyle and wellness needs of individuals and families. As an author, educator, and mother with a passion for studying and researching food and nutrition information, Sheryl works directly with clients, but also teaches workshops aimed at improving the nutritional status and overall health of participants such as her "Shop with Sheryl" classes. She is a past board member of Healthy Traditions Network, the Local Chapter of the Weston A. Price Foundation. Sheryl is married to her wonderful husband Bob and has two beautiful children Grace (twelve-years old) and Nick (eight-years-old); the inspiration for her interest in health and nutrition, and her desire to eat properly and raise a healthy family. "From my experience as a nutritionist and as a wife and mother desiring a healthy family," Sheryl says. "I recognize the importance of carefully selecting the type of food we eat, knowing where our food comes from, and buying foods in their most natural state from local farmers whenever possible."

For more about Sheryl, to get her **FREE *Healthy Handbook***, and to join her newsletter and blog community please visit her website at **www.sherylshenefelt.com**.

Join in the conversations with Sheryl Shenefelt, C.N. at:
**Facebook:** www.facebook.com/sherylshenefelt
**Twitter:** www.twitter.com/sherylshenefelt
**LinkedIn:** www.linkedin.com/in/sherylshenefelt

# Books by David Brownstein, M.D.

More information: www.drbrownstein.com

*The Statin Disaster*

Statin drugs are the most profitable drugs in the history of Big Pharma. The best of the studies show statin drugs fail to significantly lower your risk of developing heart disease. This book will tell you the truth about statin drugs. Statins are associated with a host of adverse effects including:

- ALS
- Breast Cancer
- Congestive Heart Failure
- Memory Loss
- Myopathy
- Neuropathy
- Sexual Dysfunction
- Skin Cancer

*Vitamin B12 for Health*

Vitamin B12 deficiency is occurring in epidemic numbers. This book show you the many benefits of using natural, bioidentical forms of vitamin B12 and how B12 supplements can help you achieve your optimal health. B12 therapy can treat many common ailments including:

- Anemia
- Autoimmune Illness
- Blood Clots
- Brain Fog
- Cognitive Decline
- Depression
- Fatigue
- Fibromyalgia
- Heart Disease
- Muscle Disease Neurologic Problems
- Osteoporosis
- AND MUCH MORE!

## *IODINE: WHY YOU NEED IT, WHY YOU CAN'T LIVE WITHOUT IT, 5th EDITION*

Iodine is the most misunderstood nutrient. Dr. Brownstein shows you the benefit of supplementing with iodine. Iodine deficiency is rampant. It is a world-wide problem and is at near epidemic levels in the United States. Most people wrongly assume that you get enough iodine from iodized salt. Dr. Brownstein convincingly shows you why it is vitally important to get your iodine levels measured. He shows you how iodine deficiency is related to:

- Breast cancer
- Hypothyroidism and Graves' disease
- Autoimmune illnesses
- Chronic Fatigue and Fibromyalgia
- Cancer of the prostate, ovaries, and much more!

## *OVERCOMING ARTHRITIS*

Dr. Brownstein shows you how a holistic approach can help you overcome arthritis, fibromyalgia, chronic fatigue syndrome, and other conditions. This approach encompasses the use of:

- Allergy elimination
- Detoxification
- Diet
- Natural, bioidentical hormones
- Vitamins and minerals
- Water

## *DRUGS THAT DON'T WORK and NATURAL THERAPIES THAT DO, 2nd Edition*

Dr. Brownstein's newest book will show you why the most commonly prescribed drugs may not be your best choice. Dr. Brownstein shows why drugs have so many adverse effects. The following conditions are covered in this book: high cholesterol levels, depression, GERD and reflux esophagitis, osteoporosis, inflammation, and hormone imbalances. He also gives examples of natural substances that can help the body heal.

See why the following drugs need to be avoided:

- Cholesterol-lowering drugs (statins such as Lipitor, Zocor, Mevacor, and Crestor and Zetia)
- Antidepressant drugs (SSRI's such as Prozac, Zoloft, Celexa, Paxil)
- Antacid drugs (H-2 blockers and PPI's such as Nexium, Prilosec, and Zantac)
- Osteoporosis drugs (Bisphosphonates such as Fosomax and Actonel, Zometa, and Boniva)
- Diabetes drugs (Metformin, Avandia, Glucotrol, etc.)
- Anti-inflammatory drugs (Celebrex, Vioxx, Motrin, Naprosyn, etc)
- Synthetic Hormones (Provera and Estrogen)

## *THE MIRACLE OF NATURAL HORMONES, 3rd EDITION*

Optimal health cannot be achieved with an imbalanced hormonal system. Dr. Brownstein's research on bioidentical hormones provides the reader with a plethora of information on the benefits of balancing the hormonal system with bioidentical, natural hormones. This book is in its third edition. This book gives actual case studies of the benefits of natural hormones.

See how balancing the hormonal system can help:

- Arthritis and autoimmune disorders
- Chronic fatigue syndrome and fibromyalgia
- Heart disease
- Hypothyroidism
- Menopausal symptoms
- And much more!

## *SALT YOUR WAY TO HEALTH, 2nd Edition*

Dr. Brownstein dispels many of the myths of salt—salt is bad for you, salt causes hypertension. These are just a few of the myths Dr. Brownstein tackles in this book. He shows you how the right kind of salt—unrefined salt—can have a remarkable health benefit to the body. Refined salt is a toxic, devitalized substance for the body. Unrefined salt is a necessary ingredient for achieving your optimal health. See how adding unrefined salt to your diet can help you:

- Maintain a normal blood pressure
- Balance your hormones
- Optimize your immune system
- Lower your risk for heart disease
- Overcome chronic illness

## *OVERCOMING THYROID DISORDERS, 3rd Edition*

This book provides new insight into why thyroid disorders are frequently undiagnosed and how best to treat them. The holistic treatment plan outlined in this book will show you how safe and natural remedies can help improve your thyroid function and help you achieve your optimal health.

- Detoxification
- Diet
- Graves'
- Hashimoto's Disease
- Hypothyroidism
- And Much More!!

## *THE GUIDE TO HEALTHY EATING, 2nd Edition*

Which food do you buy? Where do you shop? How do you prepare food? This book will answer all of these questions and much more. Dr. Brownstein co-wrote this book with his nutritionist, Sheryl Shenefelt, C.N. Eating real, whole foods is the most important thing you can do for your health. This book contains recipes and information on how best to feed your family. See how eating a healthier diet can help you:

- Avoid chronic illness
- Enhance your immune system
- Improve your family's nutrition

## *THE GUIDE TO A GLUTEN-FREE DIET, 2nd Edition*

What would you say if 16% of the population (1/6) had a serious, life-threatening illness that was being diagnosed correctly only 3% of the time? Gluten-sensitivity is the most frequently missed diagnosis in the U.S. This book will show how you can incorporate a healthier lifestyle by becoming gluten-free.

- Why you should become gluten-free
- What illnesses are associated with gluten sensitivity
- How to shop and cook gluten-free
- Where to find gluten-free resources

## *THE GUIDE TO A DAIRY-FREE DIET*

This book will show you why commercial dairy is not a healthy food. Dr. Brownstein and Sheryl Shenefelt, C.N., will provide you the information you need to become dairy-free. This book will dispel the myth that dairy from pasteurized milk is a healthy food choice. In fact, it is a devitalized food source which needs to be avoided.

Read this book to see why common dairy foods including milk cause:

- Osteoporosis
- Diabetes
- Allergies
- Asthma
- A Poor Immune System

## *THE SOY DECEPTION*

This book will dispel the myth that soy is a healthy food. Soy ingestion can cause a myriad of severe health issues. More information can be found online at: www.thesoydeception.com. Read this book to see why soy can cause:

- Allergies
- Cancer
- Osteoporosis
- Thyroid Disorders
- A Poor Immune System
- And, Much More!

## *THE SKINNY ON FATS*

*The Skinny on Fats* was written to educate you about the importance of consuming good sources of dietary fat. You will learn why saturated fats and cholesterol are not the enemies and why trans-fats and processed vegetable oils are the real fats that need to be avoided. This book will teach you why we need fat and why we can't live without it. Good sources of dietary fat can:

- Prevent heart disease
- Promote weight loss
- Improve the immune system
- Help prevent chronic illness

# DVD's of Dr. Brownstein's Latest Lectures Now Available!

*DVD: Iodine–The Most Misunderstood Nutrient*

*DVD: Overcoming Thyroid Disorders*

*DVD: Drugs That Don't Work and Natural Therapies That Do*

*DVD: Holistic Medicine for the 21st Century*

*DVD: Salt Your Way to Health*

*DVD: The Miracle of Natural Hormones*

*DVD: The Soy Deception*

*DVD: The Guide to a Gluten-Free Diet*

*DVD: The Guide to Healthy Eating*

## Call 1-888-647-5616 or send a check or money order *BOOKS $18 each!*

Sales Tax: For Michigan residents, please add $1.08 per book.

| **Shipping :** | 1–3 Books: | $5.00 |
|---|---|---|
| | 4–6 Books: | $4.00 |
| | 7–9 Books: | $3.00 |

**Order 10 or more books: FREE SHIPPING!**

**VOLUME DISCOUNTS AVAILABLE.**
CALL 1-888-647-5616 FOR MORE INFORMATION

**DVD's of Dr. Brownstein's Lectures Available!**
DVD's: $25.00 each

**INFORMATION OR ORDER ON-LINE AT:**
WWW.DRBROWNSTEIN.COM

You can send a check to:
**Medical Alternatives Press**
4173 Fieldbrook
West Bloomfield, MI 48323